RELIEVING PAIN

RELIEVING PAIN

A Basic Hypnotherapeutic Approach

DONALD W. SCHAFER, M.D.

JASON ARONSON INC.
Northvale, New Jersey
London

This book was set in 12-point Schneidler by TechType of Upper Saddle River, New Jersey, and printed and bound by Book-mart Press of North Bergen, New Jersey.

10 9 8 7 6 5 4 3 2 1

Library of Congress Cataloging-in-Publication Data

Schafer, Donald W.
Relieving pain : a basic hypnotherapeutic approach / by Donald W. Schafer.
p. cm.
Includes bibliographical references and index.
ISBN: 1-56821-481-2 (alk. paper)
1. Hypnotism – Therapeutic use. 2. Pain – Treatment. 3. Analgesia.
I. Title.
RB128.S33 1996
616'.047 – dc20 95-21426

Manufactured in the United States of America. Jason Aronson Inc. offers books and cassettes. For information and catalog write to Jason Aronson Inc., 230 Livingston Street, Northvale, New Jersey 07647.

I dedicate this book to my wife of 53 years, Viola, whose help and support made it possible for me to begin, work on, and finish this exciting adventure into a new career as a writer.

Contents

Foreword

I first met Donald Schafer at the 7th International Congress of Hypnosis in Philadelphia in July 1976. We were on a panel together on the use of hypnosis with burn patients. Pain is the most dreaded consequence of sustaining a serious burn. Don spoke of his work on the wards with long-standing burn pain, and I presented my approach in the emergency room using early hypnosis as a pain preventive measure. We took our wives to an elegant dinner at La Panetiere, and it was the start of an abiding friendship. Since then we have taught together at many workshops, sharing our experiences, strategies, and insights about hypnosis.

This book is different from most treatises on pain. It is written from the perspective of a psychiatrist who is using hypnosis to deal with the painful disorders of daily medical practice. Many physicians in daily medical practice, but without specialty training in psychiatry, have come from the opposite direction, and sought out hypnosis as a simplified way to add psychic care to standard therapy. The author's perspective emphasizes the *suffering* aspect of pain, and the way the mind interprets nociceptive and emotional information. This leads to a nontraditional classification of the pain syndromes, and a more rational hypnotic strategy for treatment.

Schafer emphasizes several issues that set hypnosis apart from other pain treatment modalities. He notes that there is no predictive test (including tests of hypnotizability), and so hypnosis is worth a try with any pain patient. Seldom noted in the pain literature is the effect of the American work ethic in compensable cases. Just as a sincere person believes you should give a good day's work for a day's pay, some chronic pain patients who stand to be compensated and unresponsive to therapy until it's made clear to the subconscious mind in trance that just because they are going to be paid for pain doesn't mean they must keep on having it to earn it.

Some of Don's therapeutic maneuvers seem naively simple, and one wonders if they really work. Much is made in the hypnotic literature of the importance of belief on the part of the patient, but little about the therapist. In 1 Corinthians 14:8 the Bible says, "For if the trumpet give an uncertain sound, who shall prepare himself to the battle?" Regarding hypnosis, Emil Coue

(1923) said, "Conviction is as necessary to the suggester as to his subject." It is this conviction, this faith, that enables him to obtain results where "all other means have failed." Donald Schafer believes that his patient can do this, and he imparts his confidence to them, mobilizing their own ability to do these simple maneuvers. We can all do it, too, if we can avoid giving an "uncertain sound."

Dabney M. Ewin, M.D.
Clinical Professor of Surgery
and Psychiatry
Tulane Medical School
New Orleans, Louisiana

Preface

For many years I have tried to understand and treat patients who come to me with pain as the principal symptom of an illness. My first contact with pain patients (after medical college and the army as a general medical officer in World War II) was as a general practitioner in the Midwest. After deciding to specialize, I have practiced in Southern California as a psychiatrist with a special interest in hypnotherapy and teaching hypnosis to other therapists. Through my use of hypnotherapy, I feel that my knowledge of pain has advanced beyond what is covered in most books on the subject. I hope this knowledge, which I impart here, will add to the health professional's understanding of pain. When patients have pain and can understand it with the help of their doctors, their anxiety and worry lessens. Thus, patients become better partners in the doctor–patient relationship. If families and loved ones also understand why the patient is experiencing pain, the patients will be treated much more sympathetically and empathically. Preparation for their future will also be more realistic.

I do not castigate the medical thinking appropriate to acute illnesses. Instead, I favor modifying that thinking to apply to chronic illnesses where acute thinking prevents understanding chronic conditions. Most problem pain patients fall in the category of the chronic illness. This book will help physicians expand on their tools for treatment. Just because someone has a chronic illness, with or without pain, does not mean that s/he does not deserve our best physical examinations. After all, the patient could present with symptoms of an acute illness in addition to a chronic one. Physicians should be the best doctors that they can be.

There are two appendices at the end of the book. Appendix A explains the complexity of hypnosis and why I feel a definition can never be possible in this multivariable situation. Appendix B supports my approach to clinical research in hypnosis in which is embedded my concepts of the clinical quotient. Appendices A and B are presented for those readers interested in further understanding hypnosis and for those clinicians interested in a better understanding of hypnotherapy.

This book about pain is the fruit of my labors for the last 52 years. Pain should never be considered generic, but instead should be a pain experienced in a certain place in a certain patient or client, in a certain milieu and caused by a comprehensible situation.

Acknowledgments

I wish to thank my wife, Viola, for her encouragement as well as for her editorial skills to make this book not only correct but readable. Knowing me these many years, she often knows what I mean even when I don't. Her background as a registered nurse as well as a college English teacher was invaluable in helping bring this work to fruition. I must also acknowledge the help and encouragement of our daughter and son and their spouses. Jason Aronson's staff furnished excellent help. I additionally wish to thank my brother, Lt. Gen. George E. Schafer, Medical Corps, U.S. Air Force (Retired) for his very constructive help, and Chris Backstrand, my computer tutor, for keeping my system working and for teaching me about my machine. I thank my many friends for their criticisms, comments, and support. Finally, many thanks to my patients, those I have helped control pain and those I have taught to help themselves. Working with my patients has been a continuing education in the understanding of pain. Last and certainly not least, I would like to thank my good friend and colleague Dabney Ewin, M.D., for his foreword to this book.

1

MY PERSONAL PERSPECTIVE

My experiences as a medical officer during World War II and immediately after as a general practitioner for six years gave me hands-on opportunities to deal with pain situations in the conventional ways of those times. As a practicing psychiatrist who was very interested in the use of hypnosis, I treated patients whose pain was associated with cancer. Most of these patients were terminal, which I found quite upsetting. I decided to have only three such patients at a time in my practice in order to limit the stress I felt in treating them. The hypnotherapeutic situation resulted in these patients becoming "friends." Each death, which was inevitable, was the loss of a friend.

In 1968 I joined the faculty of the California College

of Medicine at the University of California, Irvine (U.C.I.) and began a teaching career. My largest block of experience, and thus my greatest insight into this area of pain, was developed during my years in the Department of Psychiatry and Human Behavior at this college. For seven years before retirement from full-time teaching, I was the founder and director of the Hypnotherapy and Pain Evaluation Center, a part of the Psychiatry Outpatient Clinic, of which I was also the medical director. Unfortunately, that pain center has not existed since my retirement in 1984. It was then that Dr. Heidenrich and I (see Appendix B) studied the lack of correlation between depth in hypnosis as observed on the Orne-O'Connell Scale as compared with the Harvard Group Scale of Hypnotic Susceptibility.

While I was the director of that facility, the organization of the U.C.I. Medical Center demonstrated one of the problems in the approach to pain that is found in many medical establishments—*fragmentation*—in that there were pain clinics at my Hypnotherapy and Pain Evaluation Center, at the Department of Anesthesiology, and at the Department of Physical Medicine and Rehabilitation. In retrospect, each clinic seemed unaware of the activities of the others, which was unfortunate.

Since retirement from the university, my private practice consists of numerous pain patients who are referrals from other physicians. Some of my colleagues see me as a "court of last resort."

We seem to be in an era of revolutions. In addition

to the industrial one, there was a medical revolution–from the medicine-man or shaman, to the barber surgeon, to the era of sulfa-drugs, penicillin, and other agents, to the post–World War II era of steroids, antibiotics, anticancer medications, advances in modern anesthesia and surgery, and the antianxiety and antidepressive medications that are changing my specialty of psychiatry.

At this point in the modern medical revolution most physicians are still practicing "acute medicine." The revolutionizing wonder is that we have conquered most areas of acute medicine and have extended the average life expectancy by almost thirty years. We must now conquer the chronic diseases–psychoses, the autoimmune illnesses, cancer, and chronic pain–and we cannot do so if we think only "acutely." I believe there is no "generic" pain or just plain pain. There are reasons for pain and pain patients are treatable, more so if they have some understanding about their condition.

This book deals with those syndromes where pain is the dominating symptom–often with no known physical and/or biological causes. Those syndromes where pain is only one symptom of a fairly well-known condition are dealt with briefly in chapters about the general aspects of acute pain and its treatment/control. But this book focuses on chronic conditions where pain is the predominant complaint. I also discuss hypnotherapy, both as a way of understanding the psyche and as a tool for control of pain.

The guiding philosophy of my experience with

pain patients is that no one should have to hurt. Once the pain picture is complete, the victim of pain should be able to find relief. There is always a cause for pain; if it is not in the soma, it is in the psyche.

My interest in the subject of pain began while I was in medical college, when I read W. K. Livingston's (1943) book on pain. He was concerned with pain that seemed to be originating in the autonomic nervous system. He wrote of *causalgia* (now known also as reflex sympathetic dystrophy), phantom limb pain, and some aspects of intractable pain that he found could be treated by approaching the sympathetic ganglia along the spinal column. At that time this was a novel idea, but it is now the standard approach of most physicians who have patients with these conditions.

The next era in my personal evolution leading to a greater understanding of pain involved my study of hypnosis in the mid-1950s, after I had become a practicing psychiatrist. I learned that a direct suggestion to a person in hypnosis to control pain works in only a small number of pain patients: terminal cancer patients, and patients with acute organic pains caused by trauma, both accidental and as a result of surgery. It does not affect most chronic pain other than in cancer.

This book, therefore, contains the story of my "obsession" with the problem of pain and of my interest in hypnotherapy. I will emphasize hypnotherapy not only as direct suggestions to control a symptom of, or leading to, pain but also as a tool to explore and understand the pain patient during his/her treatment so that s/he has better self-understanding.

Those readers who want to know more about hypnosis are referred to the modern texts on the subject. I shall not go into detail about surgical and neurological procedures, nor will I deal with more general aspects of psychotherapy other than when I refer to the whole patient. I propose also to emphasize the friendly and humane approach to patients and their families.

I am writing for health professionals as well as interested laymen who want to understand this subject of pain. This book is not for someone who wishes to treat all comers with diets, herbs, baths, vitamins, or anything outside of mainstream medicine. It is written especially for the physician and therapist of pain patients and those close to them, so that all patients can feel healthier, understand their condition more fully, and have a better relationship with their doctors. I encourage anything that will help patients and their families feel and cope better.

This book contains some new approaches based on my experience in both physical and psychological medicine. I discuss the lesser known pain syndromes, and I offer my own unproved, but practical, classification of pain in three categories – acute, acute recurrent, and chronic. The last category is divided into the chronic-logical and the chronic career-pain patient.

> In 1960, I had a patient who opened my eyes about the complexity of pain. Mighty Little Joe was a skyscraper plumber. He enjoyed strutting around at the topmost areas, much to the admiration of other construction workers. He was 44 years of age,

white, and married. While driving home from work one evening, a truck came out of nowhere and hit him. Before impact, he had only an instant to turn his car away. The truck pushed his car across several sets of railroad tracks; each track caused his head to bang forcefully against the roof. I first saw him several months later when he was referred to me for pain control with hypnosis. He stated that he had very severe headaches as well as neck aches, which interfered with all activities. Problems in eating, sex, walking, and sleeping were a few of his complaints, and he was unable to go above the first floor of any construction site. Since he could not work, he was in litigation to be compensated for his loss.

This treatment situation occurred many years before the recognition of the syndrome now known as posttraumatic stress disorder. I used hypnosis with direct suggestion and was able to lessen his pain by 60 to 70 percent, which at least helped with many of his symptoms, but not enough to allow him to return to work. I even hospitalized him for ten days during which time I tried extended sessions in an attempt to have him go "deeper." I tried intravenous Sparine, amytal, amytal with benzadrine – all with no additional success. Other than the effect of the direct suggestion and seeing him frequently in my office at his request because I was helping him "so much," I accomplished nothing more. He only maintained the above progress until his trial, and I never saw him after the trial.

Through this case I learned about traumatically caused pain that turned into chronic pain, which seemingly was relieved after the litigation.

I have learned a great deal since then and I want to pass this knowledge on to the reader. If I can help practitioners revamp their concepts of pain so that even only one patient or client is helped, this work will not have been in vain. That there is much more to learn is self-evident. However, it cannot be accomplished by looking at the patient as just a body with a set of nerve tissues or as just a mind. Even the literature is dichotomized into organically oriented scientists and psychologically oriented scientists. We must merge and cooperate for the sake of patients experiencing pain.

2

PAIN: ACUTE VERSUS CHRONIC

As a starting definition, pain is a noxious sensation. It is also an emergency signal that something has happened, or is happening, to the physical integrity of the individual. Furthermore, pain, either acute or chronic, is always subjective or personal. Only the individual can measure pain. However, that individual is quite consistent in self-evaluation of that pain. No doctor has a test or scale by which to measure it other than the patient's subjectivity. Evaluating it is still an art, not a science. If a patient can give the doctor an idea of how the pain feels and how it changes at different times, the doctor is in a better position to diagnose and offer the best treatment.

There are physical signs of acute pain found especially in the autonomic nervous system functions as shown in the blood pressure, pulse rate, pupil size, sweating pattern (especially of the hands), and in muscle tension. There are also decreases in the flow of saliva, intestinal motility, and the flow of blood through the capillaries. There is an increase in oxygen need and blood sugar, and there is a release of adrenalin. There are emergency responses with enhanced aggression and/or defense. The anxiety surrounding the trauma increases the pain at least until that anxiety is alleviated with reassurance and/or medication. Alexithymia (from the Greek, *a* = without, *lexi* = words, *thymia* = pain) is the term applied to a small group of patients who have great difficulty putting their symptoms into words. These patients know something is wrong, but cannot find the right words to describe it. It is as if the different words for pain have vanished. In a sense, the physician has to read between the lines to be able to make a proper diagnosis. In early articles on this subject, these patients were considered to be incapable of gaining psychological insight into their conditions, but I find that it is not an all-or-none condition. I also find that these patients are hypnotizable and can be helped with that modality if suffering from acute pain, even in the emergency room. However, in a sense the physician must practice veterinarian-like medicine. This can be very frustrating to the involved medical personnel when a seemingly intelligent person is unable to describe his/her condition.

It is important not to confuse the words *pain* and *suffering*. Suffering usually accompanies pain and reveals the patient's personal experience of that pain and its meanings. Suffering with or without pain implies an emotional interpretation of the life situation. There are many kinds of suffering that do not include pain of a physiological nature. The interplay of these two words is especially important to consider in the chronic conditions. For example, many chronic, career-pain patients are suffering, but the actual physiological pain may be minimal. Suffering should probably be considered to be in the psyche and pain in the soma. However, in almost all cases, it is a combination. Chronic pain also implies at least some depression as well as anger and despair. These can be both causes, as well as results, of the ongoing pain. This pain is egocentric and usually causes agitation; the patient is often hypochondrical. This will manifest itself in psychological testing, especially on the Minnesota Multiphasic Personality Inventory. Finally, the pain behavior is often exaggerated in the chronic, career-pain patient. This can be diagnostically very helpful. Many patients with chronic-logical pain do not appear to be suffering to the extent seen in the chronic, career-pain patient.

In this book, I am dealing only with "pure" pain, which is both physical and subjective. I am not dealing with the way we often refer to a painful emotional experience. This "pure" physical pain can be divided into two groups: acute (with acute recurrent) and chronic. A clear understanding of their differences is important, for there is much more involved than the actual duration of the pain and the nerves. Acute pain is simply here and now – it did not exist before something happened, such as an injury. It must be distinguished from acute, recurrent pain and chronic pain, both of which can occur over months and even years. In acute pain, the symptom of pain may itself be the central focus for treatment. After the removal of an appendix, there is no doubt of the cause of the pain, and the pain itself can be treated with appropriate amounts of narcotics for the few days that it is needed. However, in many chronic pains, regardless of their origins, there are often no measurable physical changes, as such. Therefore, *the whole person must be treated.* Acute, recurrent pain includes most of the psychosomatic conditions in which there is pain, such as migraine and colitis.

Acute bodily pain is not a single specific kind of experience; thus, it can be described in numerous ways. Patients complaining of pain use such words as *dull, sharp, smarting, piercing, cutting, knifelike, burning, cold, throbbing, prickling, blinding, pressing, crawling, pulling,* and *lightning-like.* Patients also use terms that imply pain or near pain, but that somehow are not the same. Words such as *ache, sore, stiff,* and *itch* are examples; but for many people these words are synonymous with pain. Also, most of these words mean different things to different people in different cultures. For all of the descriptive words about pain, see *The McGill Pain Questionnaire: Major Properties and Scoring Methods* (Melzack 1975).

A person's pain threshold is that point at which an increasingly obnoxious stimulus is noticed and experienced as pain. Individuals have different thresholds of pain. Thresholds vary not only from person to person, but also from situation to situation, and within the same person at different times. However, their subjective evaluation is consistent. The patient is more aware of pain during the overnight hours when there are few distractions. A person who is very tired will notice pain that might not be noticed when rested and in a better mood.

Acute pain is a signal for the individual to do something. Cannon (1929) in his work at Harvard, further defined pain as a signal for "fight or flight." Generally speaking, acute pain follows the usual nerve pathways, similar to the way a telegraph works from the point where it originates, followed by a series of relays to the central nervous system, then another series of relays that starts the response (the "fight or flight" activities). In contrast, chronic pain usually does not follow these pathways. This is often misleading to physicians who do not differentiate between acute and chronic pain except by the length of time the pain exists.

As stated, acute pain results from some kind of a direct tissue insult to the well-being of an individual. The pain signal follows the course of the peripheral nerve up into the spinal cord, going through and crossing over in the substantia gelatinosa (Figure 2–1) into the ascending spinal thalamic tracts (the minor one may not cross and the crossover may not take place for several segments). It goes through several areas of the thalamus, then to other areas of the cortex as well as to the limbic system (an area of the brain especially involved with our emotions) for interpretation. Memory,

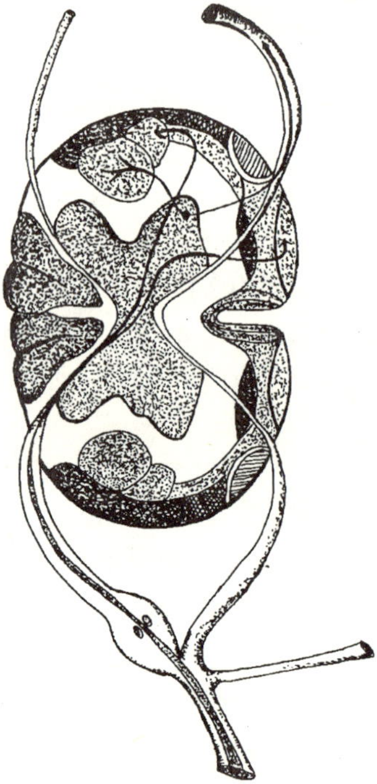

Figure 2–1. Cross Section of the Spinal Cord.

This is a schematic but incomplete lateral spinal-thalamic (LS-T) tract. This bundle of nerve fibers carries sensations of pain as well as touch from the point of an acute injury on the other side of the body to the thalamus, where it is then relayed to other parts of the brain for interpretation. Its fibers enter the spine via the ventral horn and cross over via the anterior commissure. The gray matter of the anterior and posterior horn contains the substantia gelatinosa where some of the gate theory action takes place. The ventral spinal-thalamic (VS-T) tract carries some sensations of pain as well as touch from the same side of the body to the thalamus for further distribution to other parts of the brain for interpretation. The lateral pyramidal (LP) tract is one of the pathways from the brain down to other parts of the body to activate whatever needs to be done to cope with the injury, fight or flee. The sympathic trunk is a chain of ganglia or nodes that lies outside the spine and runs alongside the vertebrae. It constantly interconnects with itself and also some of the tracts in the spine. This is a large part of the autonomic nervous system, which regulates many of the processes of the internal organs and blood vessels automatically with interplay with the limbic system, the reticular system, and others. Some types of pain are associated with this system.

emotion, and logical action then stimulate certain reflexes that may be called into play along the way. On interpretation, the person makes the decision about what to do about this pain, and then sends appropriate signals via the descending tracts.

After the "fight or flight" decision (something that is done immediately and often automatically), what can be done about the pain, especially before treatment is started? Through my use of hypnosis with many patients, I have learned that reassurance is the first step, but it should not be false. It is helpful to tell the patient that proper attention and treatment will be furnished soon. At the same time, the patient can be asked/told to relax as much as possible. A very helpful suggestion that works for nearly all of my patients is to visualize some safe and pleasant situation. This can be a nice experience from childhood or even an imaginary one. We can understand the results as due to the hypnoidal activity, even if hypnosis was not formally induced. Additionally, the patient can try to compartmentalize, to put the pain in a box.

Finally, since the frame of mind influences one's experience of pain, it is important to allay panic by trying to have the patients concentrate on staying calm, especially when they know that help is on its way. The more upset patients become, the more their muscles become tense, the more adrenalin is pumped into the system, the more they bleed, and the more they panic. This vicious cycle should be stopped if at all possible.

A fascinating case example was related to me by one of the psychology trainees working with me in

> the Hypnotherapy and Pain Evaluation Center at U.C.I.M.C. This young woman was driving home late at night with a friend when she spotted something at the side of the road. Stopping the car, she found a woman writhing in pain from a hit-and-run accident. My student placed her hand on the woman's shoulder and said, "Let me have your pain in my arm so that you can be at ease." The woman immediately relaxed and seemed comfortable. The paramedics arrived and then a complication arose. When she was asked where she hurt, her answer was that she did not hurt. My student immediately "gave her back her pain." When the patient's condition had been evaluated and she was being put in the ambulance, my student again placed her hand on the woman's shoulder. The patient was told that, "I'll keep your pain as long as needed." The woman was then comfortable.

I have observed that many patients are in an *altered state* after an injury. I would estimate that half of the patients in an emergency room are already in a trance because of both their fear and the strangeness of the setting. Therefore, reassuring suggestions and guided images are effective because the patient is already *in hypnosis*. This is even more effective if the helping person directs these ideas with his/her hand on the patient's shoulder.

This use of hypnosis or covert hypnosis is effective in the acute pain situation but usually not in the chronic. Much of this book is aimed at differentiating and explaining the differences between acute and chronic pain. In chronic pain, the therapist must always consider what is *cause* and what is *effect*. Also, many things in the milieu of the patient tend to reinforce the continuation of the pain, even if the aim is to help. Families, and physicians especially, tend to maintain patterns of chronic pain rather than relieve it. Thus, a good medical as well as psychological examination must always be done. People's reactions to pain, acute and chronic, depend on many variables.

3

THEORIES OF PAIN

There are two schools of thought about the experience of pain at its point of stimulation, both of which have some validity. The first one proposes the *specificity theory,* which states that pain is experienced as stimulation of specific end organs of the neurological system, called corpuscles or end bulbs, as well as bare nerve endings. These are therefore responsible for initiating our experiences of pain. The second, the *summation theory,* states that we are able to sense heat, cold, pressure, and sharpness, each through its own specific end bulbs. When these stimuli increase past a certain threshold, we experience pain. A combination of these theories may be helpful in understanding acute pain; however, chronic pain may or may not involve impingement on the nerve endings at the site of the original trauma, either specifically or in a summation sense, either in the present or the past.

Knowing that the experts cannot themselves agree even in their theories about acute pain, let alone chronic pain, does not help most physicians treat their patients' pain effectively. However, there is a wide difference between theories and the clinical diagnosis and treatment of pain with its many aspects.

There is, in addition, a third theory that is helpful in our understanding of pain. It was presented by Melzack and Wall (1965), who called it the *gate control theory*. Since some of their original hypothetical concepts proved to be false, there were revisions of their theory so that as it now stands, Melzack and Wall (1983) visualize three interacting systems or tracts that enable us to make decisions about fighting or fleeing.

The first of these systems has to do with rapidly conducted impulses carried from the point of injury by well-myelinated or insulated fibers to the thalamus. These impulses are forwarded to the somatosensory areas of the thalamus and the cortex, and are used for sensory discriminative purposes in order to comprehend what is happening.

The second system concerns slow conducting nerve pathways that carry almost unmyelinated fibers. These are projected to the medial reticular areas of the spinal cord, then to the brain stem and into the limbic system for motivational and emotional interpretation and reaction. These first two sets of fibers have some kind of interplay as they enter the spinal cord in what is called the substantia gelatinosa. Melzack and Wall postulated that in this area the slower fibers tended to close the gate and moderate the pain.

The third system is a central control trigger of rapidly conducting impulses that activates the neocortical or higher central nervous system processes that activate the fight or flight reaction with both unconscious and conscious aspects. With this understanding we are able to evaluate the impact of an experience in terms of our past, both as to left brain–type logical memory and right brain–type emotional memory, thereby integrating the conducting pathways for action about the pain-causing event. Through the interaction of these three systems, we are better able to comprehend our acute pains.

Pain can come from within the body as well as from the external world. An acute irritation of the appendix causes pain of the affected peritoneal area and is evaluated in the way with which most of us are familiar. We know that something is wrong with our body that we can do little about, so we call the doctor. In such a situation, we view our own body as an object (Figure 3–1).

Acute pain can be compared physiologically to panic. Both are physical conditions with increases in pulse rate, blood pressure, and muscle tension related to the amount of adrenalin released into the bloodstream. There is also increased size of the pupils, hyperperistalsis, sweating, faster breathing, and a desire to fight or flee. The responses are interlocked and feed on each other.

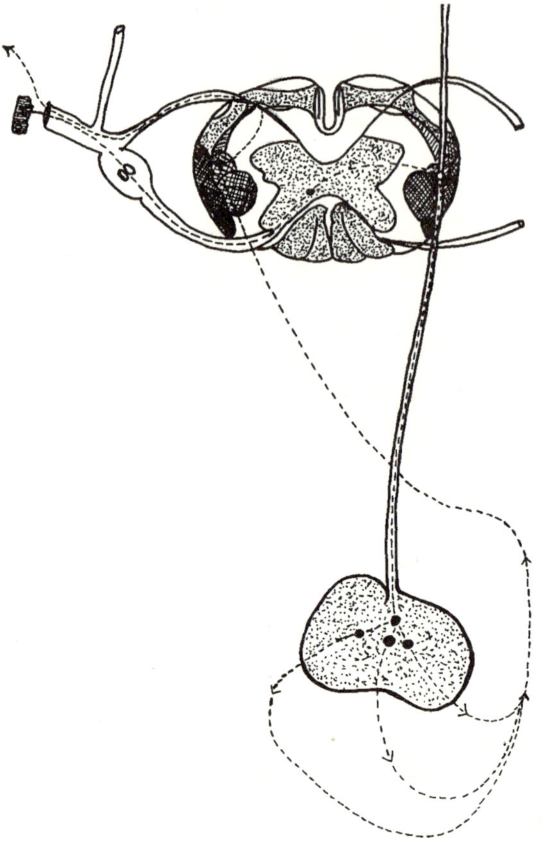

Figure 3–1. Route of a Pain Sensation and Response in Acute Pain.

This is a schematic.

1. Pain stimulus, in this case a cut to the skin, influences the pain receptor and starts the impulse up the telegraph system to the brain where it is evaluated and responds. Chemicals are released at the point of injury and influence the nerve ending or other receptor. There are really insulated and uninsulated fibers that carry the impulse at different rates all the way to the thalamus.

2. Just before reaching the spine, the nerve goes through the Spinal Ganglion where its cell body is, and then enters the spinal column at the dorsal horn. Most of the pain fibers cross through the Substantia Gelatinosa across the Anterior Commissure and into the Spinal-thalamic tract and finally to the Thalamus. There are places along this pathway that modulate the intensity of the pain. There are relay stations along the way, also. The chemical mediators in these relay stations are the Neurotransmitters.

The neurological model often does not help us understand many chronic pain conditions. This confronts many physicians with a dilemma that has resulted in reactions ranging from anger that the patient does not get well, to accusations that it is all in the patient's head. Occasionally, it results in despair in the more empathetic physicians because of their inability to help their patients. It is important to treat the whole patient if treating the symptom fails. One use of hypnosis is to see if the pain is relieved through that modality. If it is not, it implies that the symptom is not a simple *telegraph-type pain* (Schafer 1989). A telegraph-type pain is one that goes neurologically from an injured site by way of a peripheral nerve into the spinal cord, where it is relayed to other cells of an ascending nature until it reaches the brain, where it is again relayed to other cells and is finally interpreted by the injured person. Many would call this "real pain," and I believe that all pain is "real," but not all pain is neurological in origin. Hypnosis often offers relief for acute organic pain but not for most chronic pain, especially of the career type. The neurological model as discussed above in acute pain is therefore useless in most approaches to chronic pain, especially if it is not of the *logical* variety.

Chronic pain is so obviously associated with depression that the antidepressants should be tried in most chronic, benign-pain patients. The literature on pain usually does not differentiate as to which comes first, the depression or the chronic pain. Symptoms in common with the two conditions include insomnia and appetite disturbances as well as constipation or diarrhea, irritability, psychomotor retardation, orgasmic difficulties, social withdrawal, lowered pain tolerance, and somatic preoccupation.

Another way of looking at chronic pain is to separate it into three classes: (1) chronic-logical, (2) chronic recurrent (I believe this should be acute recurrent and will so place it in that category), and (3) chronic-career. Although not yet scientifically accepted as classifications, these terms are helpful in conceptualizing the patients' complaints. The *logical* variety is just what it sounds like for it is logical and understandable to physicians because of observable physical evidence.

On the other hand, the career-pain patient usually has insufficient physical and physiological evidence to account for the complaints even if the origin of the pain was logical. This patient can best be conceptualized as living in a cocoon of pain through which he rather vaguely sees his world, for the only thing in life with meaning is the pain. This in no way implies that the pain is consciously desired. It is better explained as overwhelming everything else. The recurrent pain syndromes, although usually seen as a part of a chronic disease condition, will be discussed as acute, recurrent pain, for it is not chronic, as such.

Several hypotheses help us to comprehend pain of the chronic-career type. Crue (1975) speculates about an epileptoid or seizure-like focus. Essentially he states that when pain has existed long enough and when the stimulus has gone through the substantia gelatinosa of the spinal cord intensely enough, the gate actions proposed by Melzack and Wall break down. And then the substantia gelatinosa (or some aspect of the cells in this area of the cord that involves the synapses) tends to take over. A specific group of cells can then act as an independent focus, thereby continuing to produce the pain that at first was caused by peripheral stimulation. This seems to be a useful concept and occasionally it leads to successful treatment with antiseizure medications. However, I would expand Crue's ideas to suggest that any place in these pathways, ascending or descending, where a synapse occurs might have the same epileptoid focus. This epileptoid focus could also occur in several places at the same time.

On the other hand, many psychologists and psychiatrists have looked on this type of chronic pain as a communication, even though it is of an unconscious nature. The psychotherapists Szasz (1957), Engel (1959), and Sternbach (1974) have expressly delineated this aspect of chronic pain. It was Sternbach who originated the concept of the *career-pain patient.* These writers exclude the neurological elements or at least those that promote pain in the first place. Also, generally speaking, they neglect the problem of acute pain and of chronic-logical pain.

There seems at this time to be only one source that considers both the neurological and the psychological models for pain, although earlier Szasz (1957) does mention them. In the book written for the laity by J. Blair Pace (1976) were two cartoons illustrating the psychological factors in chronic-career pain. Both show the same naked fat man facing the audience. The first cartoon portrays him like Atlas, carrying the world on his shoulders. Depressives carry the world on their shoulders. One could wonder if their character makeup predisposes them to carry such a load, which finally depresses them, or if it is the other way around. Perhaps both. The second cartoon shows him with a smile on his face stating that he would be the world's greatest lover if it were not for his bad back. How many men use this as an excuse for their lack of achievements symbolized by feelings of sexual inadequacies? Many career-pain patients suffer because of this "excuse," especially those with low back problems. They are carrying too many responsibilities and too much "emotional" weight on their shoulders, as in the first cartoon, or are defending themselves and their feared inadequacy, as in the second. I would add more cartoons that illustrate the unconscious primary and secondary gains we often observe, such as attempting to control some aspect of the world and the people in it. One can picture the bed-bound mother who rules her household with an iron fist. If anything disturbs her, it will cause her to hurt more. Everyone walks on tiptoe and jumps to please her so as not to hurt mother or feel guilty about causing her more hurt. Another aspect of these "gains" might include a person unconsciously punishing oneself for real or imaginary sins. And there is nothing more punishing than an aching back. Finally, a patient might be communicating about internal conflicts by way of the body language as expressed in one's symptom complex and as I illustrate in Chapter 6.

As a result of much research in the area of pain, *endorphins* are recognized as neurotransmitters of the pain suppressor type. They are produced throughout the body, but we are most interested in their production in the central nervous system, where they seem to have an ability to decrease the pain experience as self-produced opioids. When they were discovered, it was found that pain-controlling substances, referred to generally as narcotics, affect the same areas of the brain that produce these chemicals called polypeptides, the class name of these endorphin substances. Chronic pain is often described as occurring in people whose endorphin production systems have been exhausted. Most narcotic products do not seem to help the chronic, career-pain patients, who uselessly take a maximum amount of minor narcotics together with other substances. We have also learned that the endorphins may play a part in functions additional to pain experiences. The study of these substances, as informative as it has been, has not contributed significantly in the treatment of pain patients, especially of the chronic-career class.

The term *conditioning* is usually applied to the Pavlovian production of so-called conditioned reflexes, which need no explanation here (Pavlov 1928). I apply the term *deconditioning* as referring to a therapeutic approach to patients with symptoms that seem to have become unconsciously self-conditioned over time. Examples are migraine headaches and asthma. However most therapists doing deconditioning do not seem to conceptualize the conditioning aspect of many psychiatric and psychosomatic illnesses. I apply deconditioning procedures especially to certain habit disorders like smoking and bed-wetting as well as many phobic disorders. I also believe that the concept is applicable to many other conditions, especially of a somatic nature, where the symptom originally had meaning, either physical or psychological, but now is only a *habit* triggered by a coincidental stimulus maintained as a conditioning effect akin to the ringing of the bell for Pavlov's dogs. From a dynamic view of the unconscious, the symptom originally served a psychological purpose that now may have been resolved unconsciously even though the symptom is still present. Deconditioning this *symptom complex,* especially with hypnotherapy, is often successful. Hypnosis and teaching the patient autohypnosis give the patient not only the ability to have control, but additionally to stop the pain because it has been deconditioned. This has been effective with many of the classic psychosomatic disorders, and may be quite useful in some of the pain syndromes. If, on the other hand, the condition is still needed, or has found a new dynamic use, the application of hypnosis will not be effective, but will imply in its failure that the symptom is still needed (Schafer 1989). In many cases where hypnosis helps, biofeedback and acupuncture are also effective, regardless of the theories by which they are applied.

Chronic pain may further be understood as a third abnormal emotion. This presents a rather unique approach to what Sternbach (1974) labeled career pain. It was presented by Swanson (1984), who compared the following relationships: acute pain is to chronic (career) pain as fear is to anxiety and mourning is to depression. In each of these three conditions, the first is considered a normal emotion, while the second is pathological without a here-and-now cause. I believe that this is a breakthrough in the conceptualization of chronic pain by analogy. Swanson states that many conditions are clarified by using an analogy, even though an analogy is never exact. Whether or not a new term should be found that does not use the word *pain* is not relevant at this time but the concept is excellent, for chronic-career pain is really best viewed as an aberrant emotion.

Pain is a prominent finding in many conditions, but usually as one aspect of a disease syndrome only. When the disease is properly treated, the patient gets well and the pain is relieved along with the other symptoms. However, there are many conditions that physicians must keep in mind in making a differential diagnosis. I shall later discuss those conditions where pain is the prominent symptom. I shall also describe some conditions that may be unfamiliar to therapists treating pain. Finally, Fordyce (1976) distinguishes between certain words that may help clarify this very complicated subject. He advocates that we differentiate between suffering and nociception. The latter is what I have discussed as acute pain, with the pain of a trauma and the telegraph model, while suffering implies the more chronic form after the acute reaction is over. Suffering implies also the inclusion of many of the normal and abnormal emotions.

The acute-pain patient *hurts* and reveals this in reactions characterized by the emotional makeup of the injured person. Many chronic, career-pain patients seem to overly exhibit their pain as if they are constantly trying to convince an audience of their suffering. This does not mean that they are not suffering, but it does mean that they are not having pain of the acute type. They are also using their pain unconsciously to manipulate their surroundings through their suffering.

Since the early to middle 1980s, there has been a dearth of new theories about pain from the field of organic medicine or psychology, other than in the field of hypnosis. The most important, in my estimation, was presented by the Hilgards (1994), whose original edition was published in 1975. It has raised much debate in hypnosis circles. They proposed that the feelings of pain were not obliterated by hypnosis. Instead, the person with the pain, either in the experimental laboratories or in the clinical settings, has an unconscious or *hidden observer* that is very aware of the pain. The Hilgards have devised laboratory methods of bringing to consciousness this *other ego state* called the hidden observer to demonstrate that the patient still *feels the pain.* Other prominent workers in the field think that this is irrelevant to the clinical control of acute pain. Some theoreticians argue that the idea of this hidden observer is implanted in the subject by the suggestions of the experimental hypnotist, regardless of how carefully the experiment is performed. It is my feeling, as a clinician, that it is not important if an unconscious part of the patient's ego is aware of the pain, as long as s/he subjectively is comfortable. I also feel that there are many roads to Rome and that these concepts may be applicable to some and not others.

Many advances in the organic control of pain have

been made by anesthesiologists in their very precise approaches to patients with chronic-logical pain. Their ability to use local anesthetic agents in the involved tissues as well as in the spinal canal is an art form they have used and are perfecting even further. The patients must be carefully chosen, for these anesthetic agents will not work with chronic, career-pain patients.

Most books on chronic pain do not help our understanding of these chronic conditions and are still using the approach that is applicable mostly to the acute-pain patient. It is as if the authors use the word *pain* in a generic sense. They are utilizing and searching for new techniques to decondition or anesthetize painful conditions with or without differentiating the specific origins of the pain, if it is in the psyche. Hypnosis, meditation, biofeedback, and other remedial approaches seem to be used when nothing else works. They are clearly lacking an understanding of the patient as a whole person.

One contribution of the last few years has to do with classification (Merskey and Bogduk 1994). Although I disagree with some of their descriptions and classifications, and I will discuss some conditions they do not mention, their book is an excellent contribution and will help standardize approaches to chronic pain. Their list is the most complete one that I have seen.

4

HYPNOSIS

Hypnosis is often misunderstood by the average person as well as by most professionals who have not been trained in its uses. Most people have some idea about hypnosis, but their ideas are inaccurate if they are based on word of mouth and on observations of its use and misuse on the stage, screen, and television, where it appears to work magically. Yellow Pages and newspaper advertisements, usually placed by hypnotists who say they are "certified" or "registered," claim to help people with habit disorders, obesity, concentration, memory, and almost anything else. The words used are chosen carefully to avoid accusations of practicing medicine or psychology without a license. But these individuals sound like legitimate health science professionals. Patients should always ask about the credentials and *licensing* of anyone who treats them. Practitioners must have at least a master's degree in psychology, or a doctorate in medicine, or dentistry, and a license. Hypnosis is a tool to be used within the expertise of the individual professional. Hypnosis is not a profession.

Trained professionals–physicians, dentists, psychologists, psychiatric social workers, family counselors, and some master's-degree nurses–agree that hypnosis is an altered "mental" state usually entered into voluntarily with the help of a hypnotist. (I prefer the word *hypnotherapist*.) I disagree with the definition of hypnosis as an "altered state of consciousness." Hypnotherapy patients don't feel that there has been an altered or changed state of consciousness, for they report that they hear and remember everything, although the results show that they have been in an altered mental state of some kind, for symptoms often change dramatically. I include in the group of therapeutic altered states not only hypnosis but also biofeedback, acupuncture, use of visual imagery, instructed meditation as well as some group phenomena influenced by "charismatic leaders."

Hypnosis, like any other tool used in the health professions, is not for all types of pain. Other approaches may offer a great deal as well. Hypnosis may even be the wrong treatment in some cases. It is often used in conjunction with other types of treatments. In expert hands, it is an excellent tool in helping relieve many conditions of pain. In my opinion every pain clinic should have an experienced hypnotherapist on its staff. Hypnosis is completely safe when used by competent therapists. However, it is not magic, nor is it a cure-all.

Definitions of hypnosis generally only describe what occurs in hypnosis. But a description is not a definition. Hypnosis is as difficult to define as intelligence, sleep, and other concepts having many variables. Perhaps we should stop looking for a "definition" of hypnosis (see Appendix A).

People in (therapeutic) hypnosis feel very comfortable and usually remember what has happened during their therapeutic trance. They may not subjectively feel any different than they did before hypnosis. The advantage of using hypnosis for therapeutic purposes is that the unconscious part of the mind is nearer the surface so that it can be more efficiently explored and directed than it would be in ordinary psychotherapy. In the hypnotherapeutic relationship, that unconscious is more malleable and suggestive than in the normal alert state. This is one of the reasons that each person in this dyad must clearly understand the goals of the hypnotherapy before the induction of hypnosis.

No one has ever taken a picture or an x-ray of the "unconscious" mind. However, the unconscious is one of the most real things that I deal with as a practicing psychiatrist. The unconscious thinks differently than does the conscious mind and with a different kind of logic. Any time there is a conflict between the conscious and unconscious minds, the unconscious "wins" with the production of psychiatric symptoms such as migraine, alcoholism, kleptomania, and many other conditions. When these two parts of the mind are in good rapport, we are symptom free.

Hypnosis is an excellent tool to control acute pain, especially pain that is anticipated. Many dentists and obstetricians continued to use hypnosis during periods of its unpopularity in the last two hundred years. The obstetricians knew, for example, that a motivated woman can usually have her baby with a minimum of discomfort, especially with hypnosis, whether that hypnosis is induced during labor or delivery or had previously been taught as self-hypnosis for that purpose. This has also been true in dentistry or other procedures where pain can be expected. I see the Lamaz method as being essentially hypnosis; it is unfortunate that many of its teachers do not understand that they are utilizing hypnosis.

Of great importance is the preparation with hypnosis of the patient facing impending surgery, for it will lessen complications, provide for a more comfortable resting period after surgery, promote healing, facilitate the return of motility of the stomach and intestines, as well as often assisting in the control of bleeding. Unfortunately, this does not seem logical in our scientific society; however, it does work, and that is why the use of hypnosis should be implemented whenever possible. For example, I recently had a patient who had surgery performed on her foot for the fourth time. Each of the operations had caused her a great deal of pain. However, as with most of my postoperative patients where hypnotherapy was employed, there was no pain. She was obviously very pleased and so was I.

I introduce the idea of hypnotherapy to my patients by telling them that my job is similar to that of an orchestra director. I do not make the "music." I tell them that the patient makes the "music" by allowing the "conductor," the hypnotherapist, to direct. The musician always keeps control. A musician could get up and walk away from an orchestra at any time, even in the middle of a concert. I have never had patients walk out of my office while in a hypnotic state, but they could if they so desired.

An *induction* is a more or less formal procedure to direct a patient into hypnosis. It can be elaborate, but a shorter and simpler approach is better. After explaining to the patient how I intend to implement hypnosis, I ask the patient to get into a comfortable position, usually sitting or lying down. Technically, it can be done standing up, but this is not very practical. Usually I ask the patient to close his or her eyes and then give suggestions to relax. While observing my patients carefully, I suggest that they go deeper. When I feel they are in the right state, I make further suggestions based on the patients' and my agreement about why hypnosis is being used. After the hypnotherapy session, I suggest that the patient come out of hypnosis, feeling alert and comfortable. I usually incorporate so-called ego supportive suggestions. In other words, I work *with* patients who come to me for hypnotherapy, and thus I have a "contract" with each individual patient.

The format of my first session with a hypnotherapy patient includes the following steps. (*Note*: All patients must be assessed as to their mental status in order to understand their psychiatric and/or psychological condition.)

1. I take a thorough history and enquire about a physical examination. For the professional who is not a physician, a good liaison with the patient's physician would be necessary. One must know as much about a patient as possible before hypnosis is induced. I ask about the patient's concept of hypnosis and previous experience with it. (See Appendix A; all patients enter their first hypnosis with the conscious and unconscious concepts that they have formed about it.)

2. A verbal contract is made with the patient about the proposed goals of the hypnotherapy, with special reference to the first trance. After the first one, the patient will then recognize what I have been explaining, and no further problems about the technical aspects of hypnosis will occur. It is necessary to live up to the "contract" to the letter; the unconscious thinks very concretely and might resist if a deviation is attempted. It is better to bring the patient out of his/her hypnosis and explain before proceeding.

3. I inquire about the patient's "haven." This is a real or imaginary situation from the past, present, or future. It must be pleasant and relaxing and, above all, safe. Some therapists refer to it as their safe place, their happy place, or even their laughing place. This may be used for visual imagery during the trance.

4. All during this introductory session, motivation is enhanced in every possible way. It is necessary to be upbeat and optimistic. I slip unconscious "hints" past the defenses of the ego. A direct interpretation will usually be resisted, but a tangential remark may find its mark. For example, in the tension neck/headache syndrome, if I jokingly refer to the boss as a "pain in the neck" and then proceed without a pause, it may sow a seed that can be capitalized on later, even without hypnosis, but especially in hypnotherapy.

5. After explaining everything about hypnosis and answering their questions, I ask patients where they will be most comfortable for their hypnosis. By involving them in this aspect of the session, their unconscious becomes more cooperative.

6. Induction: I use a very simple induction that takes about 20 seconds; the longer and more elaborate ones are superfluous, in my estimation. This is my verbatim induction: "Please close your eyes. Now focus all of your attention on your eyes and make them relax. Make them so relaxed that they just won't work. When you know that they are so relaxed that they just won't work, spread that relaxation from the top of your head to the tip of your toes and feel that relaxation go all through your body. Now just relax and let yourself go deeper and deeper."

7. For deepening, I usually use a visual image of their safe haven, getting all of the senses into the image. However, I may add the suggestion, "As

you go deeper and deeper, I'll review briefly what I know about your problem." This is a disguised suggestion that they will go deeper as I review the situation.

8. I then get into the actual hypnotherapy, with direct suggestion, regression, and other imagery that will usually contain ego-supportive suggestions and posthypnotic suggestions. One of the most valuable posthypnotherapeutic suggestions is, "Please have a dream before our next session, remember it, and tell it to me and have it contain something about what your problem is. We'll try to interpret it." I also use the intrahypnosis situation to enhance and reinterpret any interpretation that I may have made prior to a trance. If the patient has self-selected to be in deep hypnosis, s/he may not remember the posthypnotic suggestion. It is up to him/her and the unconscious. I will usually include a stereotypical future induction and dehypnotization routine such as, "The next time we use hypnosis in this office, I'll ask you to fix your eyes on a spot, and I'll count to 20. By the time I reach 20, your eyes will be closed and you'll be even deeper than you are now. Similarly, to bring you out of your hypnosis, I'll count backward from 20 and when I get to 0, your eyes will open and you'll feel alert and comfortable and good about what we have done." Since I do this with every patient who will be returning, I don't have to remember or make notes of a particular induction or dehypnotization procedure for each patient.

9. After hypnosis, I inquire about the patient's experience and answer all questions. We may plan for future sessions.

As suggested above, one aspect of this approach is that anyone who comes to my office for hypnotherapy will go into whatever hypnosis is needed to accomplish what s/he came for. If this does not happen, it is not because of a lack of hypnotizability, but rather is unconscious, psychological resistance (see Appendix B). Of course, this assumes that I am doing my part of the hypnosis properly, as well as that some other variables are not interfering, such as a fire truck going past or a personality clash between patient and therapist. Because of this philosophy about hypnotherapy, I often use hypnosis for diagnostic purposes (Schafer 1989), for even a lack of relaxation has meaning. If a patient resists going into a trance, it is for some reason, and I must understand more about that patient before I can go further with hypnotherapy. The hesitancy of the beginner hypnotherapist will be empathically noted by the patient and possibly contribute to resistance.

Hypnotherapy does not encourage dependency, as such. Dependency occurs to a certain extent in all therapeutic situations. It is intensified in hypnotherapy, as are transference and countertransference. However, the aim of hypnotherapy, as with all therapies, is to make it possible for the patient to take over his/her own independent life in a healthier manner than previously. In the hypnotherapeutic situation, self-control, with or without self-hypnosis, is an early and continuing aim.

MANEUVERS USED WHILE THE PATIENT IS IN HYPNOSIS

Preoperative Maneuver

With the patient in hypnosis, I state, "After all, you don't have to have any anxieties about this coming procedure, for you are in very good hands. And you don't have to hurt any more than absolutely necessary. You may not even need any postoperative narcotics for pain, for why should you hurt? And there is no need to bleed any more than you have to, for conserving your blood will help in your quick recovery. And you can have your intestines return to normal function just as soon as possible [after abdominal operations there is temporary paralysis of the bowels]. And you can heal well without swelling and need not have any complications so that you find that this can be a good experience." All of these suggestions are couched in a form that is called a *truism,* which is a statement that cannot be argued with. I do not say, "You will not hurt"; I say, "You *need* not hurt." This is taken as a suggestion rather subtly by the unconscious, which decides what to do about it.

Solar Plexus Maneuver

After the hypnosis induction, I ask the patients to place their hand in the pit of the stomach. I explain, "The hand is now over a bunch of nerves that are called the solar plexus. These nerves radiate out to all of the areas of the body like the rays of the sun–hence its name. These nerves act just like the timer mechanism of your car, which makes sure that all of the electrical impulses go to the right places at the right times and in the right amounts and all the other 'rights.' Similarly, the solar plexus makes sure that all the nerve impulses go to the right places at the right times in the right amounts and all the other rights, so that all of your organs work just right." I then teach them how to use this in self-hypnosis. With these psychosomatic conditions, it works a large percentage of the time. I do find insight is often necessary, especially early in the course of the disease, but that is accomplished with a short course of cognitive/behavioral therapy. Most of these illnesses can be conceptualized as being treatable in this manner. It is also the approach of choice for the nausea and vomiting of x-ray and chemotherapy cancer patients as well as the nausea and vomiting of pregnacy.

The Magic Journey for Nasal Allergies

For this condition I suggest the following: "Now, as you sit there comfortably, you and I are standing on each side of you. We are getting smaller and smaller. Meanwhile I hand you a special flashlight and I have a similar one. These not only have a nice beam of light, but they also have a magical healing ray that normalizes mucous membranes. Now we are smaller, and we jump on your knees, then to your upper lip and finally we and our flashlights are small enough that we enter your left nostril. As we go into this big cave, we flash our lights around so as to normalize all of the membranes. Now we climb up to what we doctors call the lower turbinate where we flash our beams to normalize it and of course shrink down the swelling in its membranes. Then we look over there and see what looks like an open manhole. The edges are swollen so we shine our lights on them and then look into the maxillary sinus, which looks like another room in the big cave. It is filled partially with fluid. We lean into this cave far enough to shine our light and therefore normalize all of the mucus membranes in that cave. Now the sinus can drain and heal. [This is repeated for the middle turbinate.] Now we can see the opening of the tear duct, so we slip up that duct, using our lights, and arrive in the inner corner of the eye, where we shine the lights to all areas of that eye and its membranes and glands. Now we go back down the tear duct and look up to the highest of the three turbinates and repeat as before and include the frontal sinus. Then we go back and get the ethmoid and sphenoid sinuses in the same way. Now we go back down to the entrance to the cave and march straight back into the nasal passage, shining our lights over all of the membranes until we are back into the pharynx and throat. We shine our lights onto all of the adenoid and tonsil tissue that we can see, and then all the way down past the vocal cords and into the trachea and even the bronchi. Now we come back to the other nasal passage. [I repeat the first part of this for the other side of the nose.] Now we are finished and step out on the upper lip and begin to grow. We jump down to your lap and I give you my flashlight too, for you to use to make this same journey any time that you need to and when you are in a comfortable and safe place. Now we jump off of your knees and are normal size and merge back into our own selves with you able to breathe so much better and knowing that you don't have to have any more swollen and upset mucous membranes. Thank you for letting me help you." I then bring the patient out of the hypnosis.

Migraine Maneuver

I ask the patient to consent to have a mild but definite migraine while in hypnosis. If consent is not given, then I ask if the patient could imagine one. The answer is yes. I then have the patient go into hypnosis in a comfortable chair or on a couch. After s/he is in hypnosis, I ask the patient to have (or imagine) a mild and definite migraine and to signal with the right index finger slightly elevated, that s/he is having one. I then say, "Please place your hand over the area of the migraine. Now I want you to know that your migraine headache is caused by spasm of the smooth or involuntary muscles in the walls of the blood vessels inside your head. In just a moment I'll ask you to slowly make a fist as you transfer that involuntary spasm in the walls of the blood vessels of your head into the voluntary muscles of your fist which is voluntarily in spasm. When that transfer is complete, you can let your hand return to its original position. As soon as your hand is so placed, you can open your eyes and come out of your hypnosis feeling comfortable and relaxed. I want you to practice this maneuver several times a day until it becomes a part of you. Then, if you notice a migraine starting, you can get into a comfortable and safe situation and close your eyes and place your hand on your head and repeat what I have just taught you so that you never have to have another migraine headache." This can be modified to help people with tension neck/headaches or even other psychosomatic spastic conditions in other parts of the body.

Reverse Migraine Maneuver

In conditions of bleeding, especially in hemophilia in adults or children, the reverse of the above migraine maneuver can be done. This is valuable in spontaneous bleeding conditions found in hemophilia in children or adults and in situations where a hematoma might be formed because of probable mild injury in a person taking a blood thinner. This can also be utilized for some lacerations. I have found that it works in any kind of hemophilia, not just the classic type. For instance, I used it to help a physician patient with von Willebrand's hemophilia to stop bleeding in his urinary tract. I will not go into detail because it is the reverse of the above maneuver. I start the patients' routine by having them make a fist, which is a spasm of the voluntary muscles of the hand. I then ask them to place the hand over the area of bleeding and transfer the spasm to the hurt ends of the blood vessels so that the bleeding stops.

The mother or father of a hemophiliac child who is too young to take over his own autohypnosis, could do this with his/her fist next to the child's knee as the parent talks to the child whose eyes are closed. This will usually stop the "bleed" as soon as it is noticed.

Transfer of Anesthesia

This is a good maneuver for control of pain that is acute or acute recurrent and is understood by the patient. The patient, in hypnosis, is to visualize his/her safe haven. I then say, "There is a stainless steel pan by you filled with a clear solution that is a new anesthetic agent that penetrates the skin. Now place your hand in that pan and feel the coolness of the solution, then notice your hand getting numb. When it is nicely anesthetized, please raise that hand as a signal to me that it is numb. Good. Now place that hand over the area of pain and transfer the numb feeling as I say the alphabet up to the letter G . . . A B C D E F G. When the area no longer hurts, let your hand return to your lap. Please use this maneuver whenever you need it. You will come out of your hypnosis as soon as your hand is in your lap. You can do that now." Another possibility that is similar to the transfer is a rather subtle maneuver to teach a patient to "transfer" pain to another area. For example, a headache transferred to a big toe might be easier to tolerate than in the head. Or the pain might be transformed into an emotion, a mental feeling, to distract the individual from experiencing the original pain. This would be of value for those patients who cannot further control their pain. My aim is to teach the patient to control his/her own symptoms some time after gaining insight through hypnotherapeutic exploring. With many patients this is not necessary. Some patients can be taught to make a hand anesthetic and then transfer it to the painful area. If it works, fine; if not, the therapist must understand why. This can be a step in helping a somewhat resistant patient while s/he is developing further insight.

Time Distortion

A mental status examination assesses a patient's orientation as to time, place, and person. All of the aspects of the mental status examination are manipulative in the trance state. The ability to visualize oneself in a safe haven already is proof of "place distortion," so now we can utilize time distortion as well. As a later case history will reveal, time distortion is valuable in lightning pain where distortion of great quickness is enhanced by suggestions to "forget" that the condition exists, by giving this posthypnotic suggestion: "Between attacks, you will forget that anything is wrong and you will not dread the next attack. When it does occur, it will be over so quickly that you will hardly notice it at all." Suggestions of feeling "like you did ten years ago when you didn't have the condition" will often help. Visualizing five years hence when things are well can give hope.

As written here, these techniques have been simplified. None of them occurs as fast as you are able to read them. The pace is dictated by the patient, whom the hypnotherapist is watching every second for responses. Also many phrases are repeated.

Although hypnosis may be the best treatment for many conditions, it is never simple. Other than for acute pain conditions, hypnotic suggestion is often not enough by itself. A knowledge of the workings of the mind is essential for anyone using hypnosis as a therapeutic tool. Any therapist who uses hypnosis is going to become knowledgeable about the unconscious. Again, contrary to the propaganda of the lay hypnotists (Schafer 1984c), hypnosis is not a profession; it is a tool to be used within the treatment abilities of the individual health professional.

There are other conditions that can be treated by using hypnosis, such as the removal of amnesia. Hypnosis can also be used for memory exploration, regression or progression, and dream production. These areas are beyond the scope of this book. The reader is referred elsewhere [e.g., see Bowers (1976)].

I do not believe that hypnosis should ever be used for spectacular purposes. Occasionally, it has been used as the only anesthetic for major and minor surgeries. The procedure and results are spectacular. In the past, such operations were filmed and shown to health professionals. This was impressive to disbelievers. But few patients need hypnosis for these purposes. A hypnotherapist must carefully decide if it is best for the patient or whether it is a grandstand play. However, there are a few cases where it is indicated, such as a patient who is allergic to all known anesthetic agents. Also, if a patient is known to be an excellent hypnosis subject and desires hypnosis for an operation, it can be discussed by the patient, hypnotherapist, surgeon, and anesthesiologist.

I emphatically believe that hypnosis has no place in the world of entertainment. It is exploitive of not only the subject on the stage but also of the audience. Hypnosis is a very powerful tool and should be used in the right place by a trained hypnotherapist, not for the pleasure of fun seekers. Additionally, the unexpected can occur with anyone in a hypnotic trance whether it be therapeutic hypnosis or a stage entertainment. Such an occurrence is called an *abreaction.* A trained hypnotherapist working with a patient in a therapeutic setting provides for proper care. A silent abreaction could even be induced and controlled for therapeutic purposes (H. Watkins 1980). Such an occurrence would then be of benefit for the patient. But harmful reactions could occur when treatment is administered by an unlicensed individual.

Some other phenomena seen in hypnosis as well as in nature can give us more insight into hypnosis and pain problems. These are naturally occurring events that I am able to understand through my knowledge of hypnosis. I consider some of them as being experiments in nature that seem to have trance-like states. Many hypnosis phenomena occur spontaneously and naturally in everyday life without being noticed. The hypnotherapist utilizes them for the patient's benefit and in an organized fashion if they occur during a therapeutic session.

One example of a naturally occurring phenomenon, which I understand in terms of unconscious autohypnosis, involved the lessening of the pain experience by wounded American soldiers at the Anzio beachhead in Italy in World War II. These men needed much less narcotic medication than the Italian resistance fighters, which can be interpreted as the different way their wounds were experienced by the individual victim. The American soldier experienced his wound as his honorable way out of the war and felt such relief in an autohypnotic way that he often did not need much pain killer, while the Italian resistance soldier did not have such an ending to his war and usually needed the expected amount of medications.

Successful boxers also must handle their pain in such a way that they do not allow it to interfere with their boxing. I saw one ex-boxer who had root-canal dental work done without anesthesia before he had ever heard of hypnosis. He said he learned to suppress the feeling of pain when receiving blows while fighting.

There are occasional reports of people with very serious injuries who were unaware of the injuries until some time later when the emotional intensity they experienced in the traumatic situation wore off. It would seem that the extreme emotional single-mindedness of the moment kept the injury from consciousness.

Other people may modify their pain because of their character makeup. There are also some individuals who seem to compartmentalize pain almost as if they had put it in a box. They do this automatically, or they may have been taught to do this through hypnosis and self-hypnosis. In some manner, they see their pain as being moved aside in such a way that it does not interfere with their activities, although it is still there. We know of certain impassive individuals who bear their pain without showing signs of it or complaining of it. This may be due to their character or it may be cultural.

Some individuals have learned to live with pain. Many of us in the field of hypnosis feel it is wrong to insist that our patients "learn to live with it," for it implies, in a sort of backward unconscious logic, that they must have the pain if they are to live. This may interfere with proper relief of their pain, which should not have to continue indefinitely. Finally there is the reverse of this situation of pain as described by Ewin (1980). He tells of patients who have been severely injured and are unconscious, and whose first awareness that they are still alive is when they feel pain. It is as if they are thinking, "I hurt, therefore I am not dead." Some of these pain patients continue to hurt in order to live, almost as if they would die if their pain would stop. This would be to them the equivalent of death. These patients can be helped with hypnotherapy.

One term often used when discussing hypnosis, but difficult to understand in that context, is *dissociation,* which means that certain feelings can be unconsciously split off from our consciousness. It can occur naturally, as in the case of the boxer described above, and it can be taught in hypnotherapy, if such a use is indicated.

Many hypnotherapists see dissociation as the principal aspect of hypnosis, especially in the control of pain. Olness (1989) feels that one of the goals in treating pain patients is to assist them to develop an ability to gain self-regulating skills and to make those skills a part of their personality makeup. This accomplishment usually improves the quality of their lives.

Chapter 6 discusses classic psychosomatic illnesses, which are evidence of autonomic nervous system (ANS) dysfunction where the cause lies in the psyche and the effect is experienced in the soma, which results in tissue damage, usually of a temporary nature. Although most physicians view them as chronic diseases, I refer to them as acute recurrent. The different hypnosis maneuvers that are often included in their treatment are found earlier in this chapter. It is probably due to the hypnotic manipulation of the ANS that third-degree burns can be prevented. Ewin (1976) described his experience with the prevention of third-degree burns as being a relatively simple production of a hypnotic trance and direct suggestions for the skin to heal. At the same time he has the patient visualize a comfortable past situation as well as seeing the skin as normal. He stated that the hypnotherapy must be done within three to four hours of the burn (Ewin 1986). This also gave the patient self-hypnotic control of his/her pain.

Other conditions that can be mentally manipulated while a person is in a therapeutic trance include hallucinations, delusions, illusions, and related experiences. One approach to the treatment of pain is to delude a person into thinking that there is no pain, or that it has already responded to an imaginary medication. Or a hypnotherapist can have the patient hallucinate away the pain, or have the illusion that it is now an itch, but not a pain. Much of this is semantic and depends on the views of the hypnotherapist.

As a therapist, my efforts are focused on helping people, but an unethical hypnotist could direct a person into hallucinating pain that is not there. We must, however, address the question of what happens if the opposite reaction, unconsciously but naturally, occurs in the human animal. Could pains be made worse, or more continuous and overbearing, in some individuals? This again would depend on motivation, both conscious and unconscious. For example, it is impossible to evaluate whiplash neck injuries where there is the possibility of compensation in a lawsuit. This should not imply that the victim is malingering. As an example there is the story of a bus that was rear-ended. The driver noted only four passengers in the bus when he got off to assess the damages. When he returned to the bus, it was full of passengers who were all holding the backs of their necks. Malingering is always a possibility and often cannot be proven. The opposite reaction happened to a patient I saw years ago who received a much larger settlement for his injuries than he could ever imagine. It was as if he had to unconsciously continue experiencing pain until he had earned the excess compensation.

Some patients "keep" at least some of their pain, as if they must be aware of their condition, either for themselves or to be able to keep their doctor informed of their condition. The hypnotherapist might attempt to lessen the intensity of the pain without robbing the person of that valuable symptom. Cancer patients for whom hypnosis and self-hypnosis have successfully eliminated the pain and suffering do not have a reason to indefinitely retain their pain and therefore can be more comfortable (Schafer 1984a,b). However, the use of narcotics often makes patients feel "dopey" or "fuzzy." Those patients who want to be as mentally alert as possible until the inevitable end will be helped with hypnosis as a means of easing or eliminating their pain; but there are some who would live their remaining days in a narcotic fog. Hypnosis helps only those who want to be helped.

Other factors to consider are the patient's motivation and present condition, so that the context of the therapy will be optimal (Schafer and Hernandez 1978). One patient who was just starting therapeutic x-ray treatments would not even enter hypnosis on the first three meetings with a student hypnotherapist. By the fourth session his nausea and vomiting were so bad that the head of the radiology department was going to discontinue the treatments. The patient's doctor told him he would probably die if they stopped the treatment. He then went into deep hypnosis with excellent control of his treatment symptoms.

5

THE CAREER-PAIN PATIENT

The following scenario is played out regularly in the office of many doctors: A primary physician looks at his schedule for the day and groans as he sees the name of a patient he has had for a number of years. He wonders if he has missed anything about that patient? He has examined him many times, referred him to excellent specialists, listened to his tale of woe on each visit, and given him several prescriptions each time. He shudders when he thinks of the pills this patient takes each day. But he does not know what else to do. He feels upset and angry that all of his skills are to no avail in this case. The patient, on the other hand, wonders why the doctors he has seen, and they are numerous, cannot seem to help him. After all, hearts can be transplanted as well as livers, kidneys, and other organs. Why must his back continue to hurt? In addition, his adolescent son is angry because he cannot afford to buy a car but he does not seem motivated to get a job. It is a verbal battle every time he asks his son to take out the trash; he only wishes that his back would allow him to do it. His wife continually complains about her job, her boss, their children, and him. He cannot help it if the medications only make him feel dazed most of the time. He has to take them because he would surely feel worse if he did not. And he wonders why the doctor seems upset with him; he does everything the doctor asks.

This is the picture of a career-pain patient. The doctor tries to conceptualize for the patient the spinal pathways and the areas of the brain involved. The neurosurgeon refuses to operate on his back because two previous operations have not helped and he can find no pathology. The doctor, reassured by several specialists that there is nothing wrong, has relayed this to the patient who has not understood and seems puzzled. The doctor knows that there are spasms of the back muscles, but does not know why. He has even tried to refer the patient to a psychotherapist, but the patient replies that it is not in his head and he does not need a shrink. Both the doctor and the patient, as well as the family, are at their wits' end.

The career-pain patient is an enigma to both the patient and the practitioner. Therefore, practitioners must be cautioned: It is never wise or appropriate for a health professional, whether an organically oriented physician or a dynamically oriented psychotherapist, to think of chronic pain as either organic or functional. This either-or dichotomy will show in the communications with the patient. S/he will again feel offended by "yet another professional who thinks it is all in my head." However, a therapist must, paradoxically, never lose sight of the possibility of the pain being either organic, or functional, or a mixture. This distinction is a difficult one to make. If the physician is asked if he thinks the patient's pain is all in the head, one way of handling it would be to comment that all pain is interpreted in the head, and no one can tell if someone else is experiencing pain.

Sternbach (1974) termed these patients, whose pain is the only one important focus in their life, as career-pain patients. This pain dominates the patient's life, for s/he can talk of nothing else. It is as if the patient were in the proverbial cocoon and sees the world only through this haze of pain. These patients are the bane of the physician's workday; they cannot be successfully treated symptomatically. For any chance of success, *the whole patient must be treated in his milieu.* If patients are on narcotics and tranquilizers, and most of them are, they cannot acknowledge they need the medication for reasons other than to mitigate the pain. Many of these medications alter the consciousness, with some pleasurable feeling for the patient. They have no concept that they are possibly addicted, even if only in a minor way. They are habituated. It is as if their pills are magic and something terrible will happen if they do not take them exactly as the doctor ordered. Some take this to extremes, which is typical of many borderline patients formerly diagnosed as pseudoneurotic schizophrenic (Schafer 1966). It is as if the medications are a reward for their pain and suffering. Their medications usually include a so-called minor narcotic such as codeine in some form. This, together with the minor tranquilizer usually included, must be withdrawn before effective treatment of the patient is possible. This is a difficult task for both the patient and the doctor and it sometimes requires hospitalization. However, hypnosis can help suppress many symptoms of withdrawal. Additionally, time distortion via hypnosis can also help such a patient to be handled as an outpatient. (However, some state laws preclude treating an addict as an outpatient.)

If the patient is involved in litigation, it is almost impossible to treat him until after the case is settled. The rules of industrial compensation, as well as those governing civil court actions, tend to prolong the time between the injury and the settlement so that this pain is deeply embedded and conditioned before that litigation is over. This makes the definitive treatment much more difficult even after a settlement has been made. By this time not only are the organic aspects altered, but the secondary gains (or losses) have occurred for both the patient and the family. The patient/litigant who is suffering is reacting unconsciously, for most of these patients are not malingering. The patients' unconscious processes (regardless of their loud conscious denials to the contrary) realize that a jaunty walk into a courtroom with a complaint of having had terrible pain in the recent past will have very little chance of getting just compensation. However, if they enter a court with a terrible limp or in a wheelchair and have a worried look and furrowed brow, the jury is more likely to extend "justice."

In spite of this, it is valid to test the situation with a hypnosis approach, for an occasional patient will be "cured," or at least helped, even in the presence of litigation as the case history in Chapter 1 demonstrated. However, the best time for hypnotherapy is within the first month after the injury or soon after the settlement; if hypnosis has now miraculously cured the patient, no one can accuse him/her of having put on "an act" for the court, which is primarily unconscious. The unconscious also plays a large part in gaining Social Security Insurance or private insurance benefits. The entire process rouses patients' anger when they have been put through so many examinations and evaluations, which also lengthen the time of both suffering and litigation.

An unexpected phenomenon occurs in many patients who receive ongoing compensation for a disabling pain condition. It is as if they feel they must "earn" their pay by continuing to hurt and be inactive. Many also fear being spied upon and reported if caught even just sweeping the sidewalk. This is fear, not paranoia.

Many of these patients, due to their psychological condition, find themselves in conflict over the work ethic. It is difficult for people with a strong work ethic to accept that any person cannot work in some way.

But we don't confront people with a work-or-starve ultimatum. Many unfortunate sufferers would love to be able to work. However, some of them are unconsciously unable to conceptualize working even though their physicians cannot see any pathophysiological involvement. In many cases, it is the better part of valor to correctly assess these patients as never being able to work again, but some of my colleagues disagree with me about this. From a psychological view, allowing that patient to accept a nonworking status without guilt in order to live more comfortably may be the best and most humane course to follow. Also, if pushed too hard by teams of rehabilitation examiners, some of these patients may commit suicide.

Many of these patients are living on Social Security Insurance and/or other benefits they financed by paying money into a fund while working; a gamble was made and "won"–that is how insurance works. So hasn't the patient "earned it?"

A large percentage of low back pain patients do have spasms of the back muscles. They are still considered career-pain patients, for they are not consciously making their backs rigid. The concept of cause and effect leads us to think that where there is spasm there must be pathology causing it. But that pathology need not be in the soma. This is illustrated by the following case.

A married, 40-year-old Caucasian dairy worker, three years previous to my first meeting him, had twist-lifted a large milk container and ruptured a lumbar intervertebral disk, which immediately resulted in pain that required hospitalization and surgical relief. He then felt that he returned to work too early, and three weeks later he twist-lifted another can and ruptured another disk. In spite of the pain, he continued to work until hospitalized one month later. He had another surgical procedure, but this time the pain did not cease. One year later, his coccyx was removed. Since then, his image of his lumbar spine is that each vertebra is made of a semi-solid block of mush. He was already on aspirin with 30 mg of codeine four times a day; Valium, 5 mg four times a day; and a nonbarbiturate sleeping medication (which I have changed occasionally). I added Elavil 25 mg four times a day. He is still on these medications. I saw him weekly for three years. Within my role as a psychotherapist, as a good and protecting father in the transference situation, any alteration of these medications is precluded, even though I recognize that they also act somewhat as placebos. I now see him for a half-hour every two or three months as maintenance therapy; he is not running to every doctor he hears of. He is not spending a lot of taxpayers' money on useless examinations and treatments. He is "relatively" comfortable and accepting of his life and the limitations he has to bear.

The patient's history revealed that he had an identical twin brother who was their father's favorite. When they were 5 years old, they had a severe, febrile illness resulting in the death of his twin.

Since then, the father has treated the patient as if it were his fault that only he survived, so much so that the patient's mother soon left the home. The father soon remarried and he and the new stepmother continued berating the patient until he ran away at 16. The father continues to blame the patient. The patient had just recently received another berating letter from his father.

On several occasions, the insurance company sent a team of rehabilitation experts. Following each visit, my patient became suicidal. I finally wrote a strong, and successful, letter to the insurance company objecting to this inhumane treatment. He is now fairly comfortable on the listed medications, which we are lowering slowly for both medicinal and psychological reasons. He received his settlement from the Industrial Commission. He receives Social Security Insurance benefits (I had to testify in court for him to get these benefits). His low back muscles are in fairly constant spasm; he constantly fears someone will see him walking in his driveway and that he will be forced to forgo his benefits. In the years I have known him, he has changed very little other than becoming somewhat less fearful. At the present, I do not expect any further changes to occur.

Is there any help for a career-pain patient? The above case illustrates that help was only moderately successful. The next case illustrates a good result.

A married, Caucasian disabled restaurant worker, aged 49, was referred to the University of California, Irvine Medical Center Hypnotherapy and Pain Evaluation Center because of chronic low back pain and misuse of medications. Her history revealed that she was injured by a fall while at work several years previously. Repeated examination, as well as an extended court battle, resulted in her permanent retirement on Social Security Insurance benefits as well as an industrial commission settlement.

To my surprise, no previous physician had inquired into her living situation. She had a somewhat older husband who had three previous coronary occlusions and was afraid to have her out of his sight for fear he would have another one and would need someone to call 911. They have an unmarried daughter, who is pregnant, and a son, who has a diagnosis of chronic schizophrenia and is periodically treated in a state hospital. When he is not in the hospital, he frequently comes to his parents' home and terrorizes them.

By the time she was seen by us, she admitted to a daily intake of fifteen aspirin with one grain of codeine each. We worked with her, teaching her how to handle her husband safely but in such a way that she did not feel a prisoner in her own home. Their daughter gave birth uneventfully; and, for reasons that we never understood, their son moved to another state. During this time, we were able to lower her intake of the aspirin with codeine to three capsules a day. Inasmuch as this woman was permanently retired and drawing compensation and benefits, we felt that she would never work, but must continue to see herself as disabled, which included having to take at least a minimum of medication. We therefore advised her that the three capsules a day would work better than the large amount she had previously taken. We reinforced these ideas both in and out of hypnosis. We felt that this was a point of maximum benefit and therefore a success, and it was accomplished in five visits by one of the students under my supervision.

The chronic, career-pain patient can be helped by an understanding therapist, physician, or health professional working within the framework of the patient's life. The practitioner must take into consideration the patient's life circumstances while looking for the unconscious primary and secondary gains of the pain syndrome. In this way it is possible to "outsmart" the unconscious and/or gain insight into the patient's condition. The patient's early background will often give the clues needed. It is possible to "cure" such a patient, or at least to get him/her to a point of maximum benefit with a minimum of medication and a maximum of comfort, by utilizing psychotherapy enhanced with hypnotherapy. This usually entails long-term treatment. If the use of hypnosis fails with prestige suggestions and other maneuvers, it emphasizes that the symptoms are unconsciously necessary to the patient, even if there are structural changes in the areas of pain. Use this "failure" diagnostically (Schafer 1989), for the patient is probably a chronic career-pain patient.

Continuing to search for and even treat nonexistent pathology of the soma in the chronic-career-pain patients will not only cement the patients' beliefs that their problems must be organic, but will make them inaccessible to psychotherapy, including hypnotherapy.

Crasilneck (1995) discusses his bombardment technique for intractable organic pain. At first sight, some of the patients he treated seem to have been chronic, career-pain patients. However, Crasilneck dealt with at least enough of the dynamics of their secondary gains to make them amenable to hypnotherapy. He bombards these chronic pain patients with hypnotic approaches that, to me, seemed to overwhelm them. He uses six different hypnosis procedures that include relaxation and teaching patients self-hypnosis over a ten-hour course of treatment. My hypnosis approach is more flexible and shorter. I prefer to use hypnosis more diagnostically and work with the dynamics, letting the patients take control of their own health. His patients all seem to have tried hypnosis before and failed. This bombardment may have cut through resistances set up by previous failures. However, it is results that we are after. We should always remain flexible and fit our treatment approaches to the individual patient. Crasilneck feels there is no comparison of his bombardment technique with flooding and implosion therapy utilizing hypnosis as discussed by Kroger (1977). The latter technique uses anxiety as a path to insight and cure. Crasilneck's bombardments promote relaxation.

6

ACUTE RECURRENT PAIN: THE CLASSIC PSYCHOSOMATIC DISORDERS

Although many texts place acute recurrent pain syndromes in the chronic category, I feel that they warrant their own special classification. Symptoms of this group of disorders are commonly referred to as classic psychosomatic syndromes. The most important ones are migraine headache, tension neck/headache, spastic colitis, and duodenal ulcer. Asthma, with its severe distress, should also be in this group of disorders, as should atopic dermatitis, for the itching approaches acute pain. Osteoarthritis also belongs here but will be discussed in a later chapter. Hypertension is often included in this category of illnesses but most patients can have this condition for many years without having any symptoms; I therefore do not include it for reasons clarified below. Despite some disagreement, dysmenorrhea belongs in this category. The classic psychosomatic diseases were explored psychodynamically by Franz Alexander (1950). He also included ulcerative colitis, which is now listed as one of the autoimmune disorders.

The symptoms of these multifaceted conditions can be attributed to autonomic nervous system dysfunction. The pathophysiology is probably in the smooth muscles of the walls of the blood vessels, as in migraine, or it may be the burning of acid in duodenal ulcers resulting from overstimulation of the acid-producing cells caused by dilatation of the blood vessels of the stomach as a result of overstimulation of the vagus nerve. This is usually treated symptomatically by neutralizing the acid and/or inhibiting the action of the vagus nerve. Although these illnesses are treated symptomatically with specific medications or surgery, the proper and complete treatment should also include an exploration of why the autonomic nervous system is dysfunctional. Careful attention to psychosomatic or "body" language as communication will usually yield an understanding of the dynamic unconscious conflicts. Insight will usually lead to a cure and eliminate the need of the purely symptomatic approaches, which in themselves can cause complications. Many times, regressive hypnotherapeutic explorations, the somatic bridge (Wicks 1984), will be the approach of choice, when aided by self-hypnosis maneuvers.

Patients with these disorders are communicating through a variety of channels. It is imperative that physicians be sensitive to all modes of communication. Too often, because of the pressure of time, physicians develop a mind set and hear and observe only what they expect, often in very literal terms. The language of metaphor can help in understanding these syndromes as unconscious communications. These somatic language statements include some of the following: the situation is a real "headache," what a "pain in the neck" the boss is, I just can't "stomach" that, my "gorge rises," it is "stuck in my craw," I'm really "griped" about that and I'm just "itching" to get at that, something is "rubbing me the wrong way" or "getting under my skin." These psychosomatic metaphorical phrases are found in all languages. They are often considered to be only clichés, not bodily communications, for as miserable as the individual is, metaphorical language keeps forbidden thoughts and ideas out of consciousness. Some of these phrases remain popular, while others go out of use; for example, the word *gorge* used as a noun has gone out of fashion. Many people are not familiar with the biblical use of this word, for it means the content of the stomach. "My gorge rises" means simply that something makes me want to vomit. Patients often communicate in this subtle fashion, which is not comprehended consciously by either the patient or doctor. Patients have no idea that the symptoms are a communication, for they need to keep the forbidden instinctual thoughts and feelings out of consciousness. Each psychosomatic disorder is, at the time of onset, a dynamically and unconsciously needed condition that is used as a defense in some manner.

Cheek and LeCron (1968) state that the psychosomatic disorder embodies six factors. My own list is as follows:

1. The condition is a way of bodily binding or somaticizing an instinctual derivative that cannot be allowed into consciousness because of prior patterns of rearing and conditioning.
2. This bound instinctual derivative is expressed symbolically via body language.
3. The patient is punished by the symptom complex even though the forbidden instinctual drive is not allowed into consciousness.
4. The effect of the instinctual derivative strikes its target even though no one is consciously aware of it.

As an example, Mary, a young woman, is asked out on a date, two weeks in advance, for an evening at the theater and dinner. Although she has a feeling that there is no future for her with the young man, she cannot think of an excuse and accepts the date. At four o'clock on the Saturday of the date, she suddenly suffers from one of her severe migraines. An hour later, the young man arrives at the home and is met by Mary's mother who explains that Mary has a terrible sick headache and cannot go. Mary is punished for the unacceptable feeling of anger at the young man, even though it was her choice to accept the date. This anger could not come into consciousness and had to be handled as a headache, but the target for this feeling, the young man, also was punished. The common denominator of these painful psychosomatic illnesses, the painful self-punishment in the form of this severe headache, is the most important aspect of psychosomatic diseases for all physicians to recognize. Psychotherapy is often needed for the patient to gain insight and cure.

Aggressive instinctual drives are considered forbidden in our society. They are the modern sin. One must not even think of anything hostile. I often have my patients join my "Down with Thumper Club." Thumper is the little lop-eared rabbit in Disney's *Bambi,* whose favorite remark to his mother, after she caught him saying something hostile, was, "I know, Momma, if you can't say something nice, don't say nothing at all." If a child is continually told this, hostile thoughts will finally be prevented from becoming conscious. However, something has to be done with the instinctual hostility and aggression, so psychosomatic patients turn it around onto the self with the production of their symptoms.

If the condition is of long standing, it may have become a habit or a conditioned response that the patient can easily be taught to control and soon eliminate through self-hypnosis. The specific constellation of aggressive feelings is no longer actively needed. But, as mentioned earlier, if the hypnosis does not affect this control, it may be assumed that the symptoms are dynamically needed (Schafer 1989).

MIGRAINE

There are two types of patients who suffer from migraine headaches. There are those who need the symptoms dynamically, who are usually newly afflicted, and those who no longer have that need and have not unconsciously found another use for the symptom, for it is now only a conditioned reflex. Inquiring into the patient's history helps make this determination.

When I treat migraine patients with hypnotherapy, I first explain hypnosis and then have the patient enter a trance. Having secured the patient's permission, I produce a mild but definite typical headache. I utilize what I call the "migraine maneuver" and instruct the patient in its use. Typically, two weeks later, the patient returns with one of two comments. "Gee, Doc, I had three headaches and was successful with that maneuver you taught me." With this kind of response, I continue impressing the patient with the value of the maneuver. I usually do not point out that s/he has produced a migraine and has removed it, I leave this for the unconscious to understand. It would be a waste of time to seek insight about the origins of the condition; the cure proves that the attacks are no longer needed. The migraine maneuver is described in detail in Chapter 4, along with other valuable maneuvers.

On the other hand, if the patient returns bitterly complaining of a recent migraine and I find that the maneuver was not used because it was forgotten, I take this as an unconscious message that the symptom is needed dynamically, and proceed with psychotherapy with or without hypnotherapy. In either case, the hypnosis itself has led to a quick evaluation.

In those psychosomatic conditions that are proven to be needed, we must work out the origins of the symptom complex insightfully to control the autonomic nervous system involvement. Hypnotherapeutic regression will often help find the material needed much more quickly than standard psychotherapy. The *affect bridge* (Watkins 1971) is an excellent approach to gaining insight into the early stages of a patient's life. This is also termed the *somatic bridge* (Wicks 1984). The approach will be elucidated in another chapter.

Hypnosis offers a great deal of therapeutic control over the principal purpose of the autonomic nervous system, which is to control the caliber of the blood vessels. By analogy, any dysfunction of this system can be seen as a *negative self-hypnosis,* a term used by Araoz (1985). This implies that the unconscious, which has defensively produced the symptoms, is stronger than an external hypnotherapist because the dynamics involved in the production of the symptoms are still actively needed by the patient's unconscious. Once the unconscious dynamics are understood, hypnosis easily gives control to the patient if the symptom still persists.

In treating these patients, the hypnotherapist must work closely with the primary physician, because some medications, even if no longer needed, must be curtailed slowly so as not to produce a withdrawal effect. As long as the medication is needed and helping there is no reason to discontinue it, but the discontinuance should be a stated part of the goals of therapy. A medication that is no longer needed physiologically should not be continued. (See Chapter 9 for a case example.)

Some doctors who are not familiar with hypnosis question the removal of a symptom, as if the patient is being robbed. This criticism can be responded to in two ways. First, when a surgeon removes the stomach because of ulcers, is he not robbing that patient of symptoms? Does not the prescribing of antiasthma medications rob the patient of his symptoms? I maintain that the symptom-removal approach of modern medicine is not enough, and that psychotherapy, especially hypnotherapy, is an approach that should be used, before a more drastic treatment is tried. Second, if the symptom goes away with direct hypnosis suggestion, it implies that it is no longer needed in the economy of the unconscious defenses, so it is not robbed from the patient. I have no argument with treating these conditions symptomatically if proper psychological explorations are under way so as to ensure a cure. The occasional patient who is "cured" by a symptomatically aimed medication is probably a patient whose symptoms are only conditioned ones. The conditioned reflex is broken up pharmacologically at times.

Also, modern hypnosis is permissive. The patient's unconscious will see that no hypnotherapist is going to "rob" him/her of any symptom. Efforts will be made to give the patient self-control of his symptoms. If that does not produce the desired effects, hypnotherapy will explore and again make it possible, through insight, for the patient to control the condition (see Chapter 9).

The same type of approach used for migraine patients can be used for others syndromes of the classic psychosomatic group, as described in the following sections.

TENSION HEAD/NECK ACHE

I always ask the referral source to tell me who the "pain in the neck" is in the life of that patient. Almost invariably, there is one. It is usually the spouse, a child, or an employer. I then see the patient, get the background of the illness as well as any other pertinent material, and try a modified migraine maneuver as detailed in Chapter 4. Again, if the symptom is now only a conditioned one, this maneuver will give control to the patient. Otherwise, we work on the necessary insight. This condition, along with its variant, the scalp muscle contraction headache, will be further discussed in Chapter 9.

ASTHMA

The asthmatic patient seldom complains of pain, as such; however, the patient is physically suffering. Oxygen starvation is a painful experience. Regardless of the source of the asthmatic condition, I utilize a hypnotherapeutic approach to give the patient control of the illness, as follows: "Is it all right for you to develop a mild but definite attack of asthma when in a comfortable hypnosis?" If the patient says no, which is rare, I immediately ask him or her merely to imagine such an attack while in the trance.

When the patients are in hypnosis, I again ask their permission for them to have a mild but definite attack. I request an answer with an ideomotor signal, usually raising the right index finger. They usually answer yes. I then ask them to produce such an attack and signal when an asthmatic condition is present, by raising the same finger. Usually, the attack is obvious by their breathing. I then ask them to visualize the little muscles surrounding the neck of the end bulbs in their lungs and to let them relax so that the trapped air can get out. When the patients have done this and breathing is back to normal, my instruction is to practice this while using the solar plexus maneuver (Chapter 4), which I immediately teach them to use at any time they have a need and are in a comfortable and safe place. I find that most of these patients have had their asthma for a long time and are therefore ready to be "deconditioned." However, if the maneuver does not work, it implies the ongoing need for the symptom.

SPASTIC COLITIS (IRRITABLE BOWEL SYNDROME)

These patients are "griped" about someone, or something. My questioning will include a search for the source of their symptoms. Whether that source is found quickly or not, I usually teach them the hypnotherapeutic solar plexus maneuver. As the cause of the griping pains is usually still present, psychotherapy is usually needed. However, it is still treatable mostly in the here and now, without having to do regressive hypnotherapy.

PEPTIC ULCER

There are so many body language communicative phrases about this condition, that I often use a shotgun approach by asking rather oblique questions. I do this with humorous remarks so as to "slip" a potentially insightful idea into the unconsious when the defenses of the patient are not aroused. It pays off later. I do this in other illnesses, both for pain patients and patients with other diseases. A preparatory remark will plant the seeds for later use: "I can't stomach that, or him, or her." "I'm so angry that my gorge rises." "I feel like I was just kicked in the stomach." "I feel like it's stuck in my craw." These are a few of the remarks that the body may be communicating that can be used in a joking manner to get the attention of the unconscious without alerting the unconscious defenses. Although peptic ulcer can often be helped with the solar plexus maneuver, in my experience cases of peptic ulcer seem more deeply rooted in the unconscious than most of the others and may take much insightful therapy.

ATOPIC DERMATITIS

The pattern of this skin ailment makes it fairly easy to diagnose. The inhibited anger is also fairly easy to uncover. Since the skin is involved, there is a myriad of somatic phrases that can be examined: "I'm just itching to get at someone." "It's rubbing me the wrong way." "It's getting under my skin." "It's just rubbing me raw." These patients often have a personality that is very sensitive. It is as if they are trying to grow thicker skin like a rhinoceros to protect the most sensitive areas of the skin, which is the usual distribution of the lesions. I find that insight is usually necessary. Conjoint therapy may be necessary if the spouse is the "cause."

DYSMENORRHEA

In my experience, this is a condition interwoven with the woman's unconscious ambivalence about her acceptance of herself as a female. The solar plexus maneuver often helps, especially with remarks about the value of her femininity. When she realizes that men and women are different and that there is value to both sexes in being what they are, a great deal can be accomplished. Incidentally, if we look at the tried and true treatments for severe dysmenorrhea such as dilation and curretage (D & C) and pregnancy, both disrupt the patency of the cervix, allowing the menses easy outlet, for the cervix cannot then spasm. A D & C usually helps at least temporarily.

ENDOMETRIOSIS

I find that this patient is often almost sickly sweet. Not only must she be helped to appreciate herself, but she must be taught to deal with a high amount of unconscious rage being covered by the sweet personality.

I speculate about the psychopathology as follows: This woman is full of rage, which is so forbidden that she cannot even be aware of it. Her rage is symbolized by blood, which she also does not dare show. So her cervix goes into spasm to hold the monthly menstrual blood from showing. After her pain has "punished" her enough for having her unconscious anger, even though she is unaware of the rage, the cervix can relax and her period continue comfortably. But before this happens, some of the menstrual cellular material has refluxed up the fallopian tubes and has seeded in the lower peritoneal areas, only to form cysts with each succeeding period, thereby punishing her more. Again, the solar plexus maneuver is often very helpful, and insightful hypnotherapy will make a cure possible if treated early. Menstrual period–inhibiting hormones may still be necessary until the menopause, but the condition is often ameliorated by the therapy.

ACNE VULGARIS

According to some textbooks on dermatology, one-third of treatment regimens succeed. I am not sure that this condition is a painful one, but the teen with acne is in emotional agony. I contend that most of the medicinal treatments for this condition are placebos, but they work as many placebos do. Hypnotherapy usually cures the condition with suggestions to visualize healthy skin with both a normal blood supply and nerve impulses to the aciner glands, together with remarks to stop effacing the self, and finally with a rather tangential discussion of being a defense against interplay with the opposite sex. This is generally a condition of adolescence. One or two sessions usually produce a clearing of the skin.

The classic psychosomatic diseases with accompanying pain are inadequately treated when that treatment is aimed only at the symptoms. Most of my physician colleagues reject this as a silly notion. I do not disagree with symptomatic treatment if attempts are being made to find out the *why* of the condition. In my opinion, most physicians seem content to accept just the *what.* But this *what* is not enough. We have a great deal of understanding of the endorphins and the other neurotransmitters, but we are still treating the conditions symptomatically. We must assume that there is a reason for these substances becoming abnormal. It is my opinion that most of the reason is found in the psyche.

7

CHRONIC-LOGICAL PAIN SYNDROMES

The pain of chronic-logical pain syndromes is nociceptive, in which a nerve receptor or path is involved. The term *nociceptive* is often used as a synonym for the words *pain* or *painful,* in which an actual nerve is being stimulated, as opposed to so-called functional, emotional, or career pain, in which there is no explainable neurological involvement with nerve pathways. Chronic-logical pain syndromes have been long recognized by their frequent occurrences and their lack of association with specific disease processes. I use the word *logical* because in our critical thinking this kind of pain does make sense and is therefore logical. Whether the pathology is well understood or not, the term implies a consistency of diagnosis and treatment.

REFLEX SYMPATHETIC DYSTROPHY OR CAUSALGIA, AND PHANTOM LIMB PAIN

The mechanisms that produce the pain in this category are not easily understood from a scientific viewpoint. In phantom limb and in sympathetic dystrophy (very similar to causalgia and often used interchangeably), there is organic dysfunction of the autonomic nervous system as observed in the abnormal colorations, temperature, and sweating patterns of the skin areas involved.

In the case of phantom phenomena, there is strong reason to believe that a disturbance of the patient's ego image is also involved. There is an inability of the ego to accept that a body part is missing and the psyche keeps the involved autonomic nervous system stimulated in some manner. If it hurts, it cannot be gone! Many different procedures have been devised to cope with these conditions, including progressively higher amputation to remove the phantom sensation. This rarely works, thereby disproving the idea that the usual cause is a neuroma, a small tumor of the cut nerve, made of tangled nerve fibers, and cells in the end of the cut nerve.

For sympathetic dystrophy, Livingston (1943) introduced injection and/or surgical removal of one or more of the sympathetic ganglia (an organized group of nerve cells lying next to the spinal column – see Figure 3–1). This often gives relief. However, hypnotherapy is a treatment of choice that generally works. This is particularly true in the absence of litigation or other secondary gains, which may also explain some of the failures of the surgical procedures. If hypnosis does not furnish relief, no harm has been done, whereas surgical procedures are not only expensive but also irreversible. Hypnosis will often "normalize" autonomic nervous system (ANS) dysfunctions even when organically caused.

> A 40-year-old, married, Caucasian woman was referred to me for burning pain in her right hand and arm extending into her arm pit and shoulder. Her history revealed that she had been working on a heat press machine, which caught, crushed, and burned her hand. She immediately felt a severe burning up to her elbow. She healed with very little movement possible in her hand and fingers. Her hand was frozen in what is called a position of function. It looked like a normal hand as to position and appearance, even if without motion. Causalgia and sympathetic dystrophy are manifested by complaints of severe burning sensations as well as deep aching types of pain, which this patient also had. Severe burning pain always means ANS dysfunction, in this case produced traumatically. There is usually a mottling of the skin as well as spotty areas of dryness and of perspiration.
>
> The patient informed me of two important factors: (1) she was engaged in punitive litigation with the company that had employed her because they had not corrected a known mechanical defect that led to her accident, and (2) her stellate ganglion had

been surgically removed. The latter procedure would usually be effective in a case of this nature, but instead resulted in the pain shifting to a higher point in her arm. Although I considered both of these factors, the litigation and the unsuccessful surgery, as bad omens, I agreed to treat her. After getting the history, I directed her into her hypnosis and gave her suggestions that the blood and nerve supply were now normal and she did not have to continue to hurt. Much to my surprise, at her next appointment she informed me of her "miraculous" cure. She had complete control of her pain with her own self-hypnosis by using the induction maneuver I used on her first visit. One year later, she was still doing well. This, again, may illustrate the power of the psyche. Perhaps the crushed hand was, in her unconscious, enough to demonstrate to everyone that she deserved a valid settlement.

A 22-year-old unmarried woman came to the center with a complaint of phantom limb pain. She told us that she had a bone cancer (probably a Ewing's tumor) removed at the age of 14. At relatively regular intervals, inch by inch, the leg stump was surgically shortened in attempts to relieve the phantom sensation, and it now was disarticulated at the hip. Although there was nothing left to remove, she had experienced no relief from pain. In three visits, utilizing hypnotic direct suggestions that she need not have the pain anymore and that she should accept having only three limbs, her phantom pain vanished and never recurred.

RAYNAUD'S DISEASE

Although this is a fairly easy condition to diagnose, it is included here because hypnotherapy is a first treatment of choice, as hypnosis gives excellent control and self-control of ANS problems. In this condition, with attacks of aching, burning, and feelings of coldness, and a blue cast to the extremities, which follows an initial whiteness, especially of the hands, caused by vasoconstriction of the arteries, the patient generally already has his/her diagnosis. Wearing gloves and other warming maneuvers gives only temporary relief. With hypnotherapy, the ANS dysfunction is usually sufficiently controlled that searching for causes is unnecessary. The disease predominates in females by a ratio of 5:1, and generally strikes between the ages of 10 and 40. Emotional stress and the onset of the menses are two recognized triggers. Teaching self-hypnosis usually gives the patient control. Visualizations of being warmed by the sun or of having hands in warm water can be added to the patient's visualizations during self-hypnosis. Only a few treatments are necessary in most patients. The younger the patient, the quicker the condition is overcome. Sympathetic blocks help temporarily, and sometimes calcium channel blocking agents also help. However, hypnosis is the treatment of choice. A similarly appearing condition is called Raynaud's phenomenon and is a symptom of certain rare disease states. Again, careful history and physical examinations are necessary.

ACROCYANOSIS

This persistent blueness alternating with whiteness and coldness of the hands and feet is mentioned here because these patients are uncomfortable and often complain of aching pain. They are miserable in cold weather. This condition starts in late childhood and seems to have a hereditary background. It is easy to confuse with Raynaud's disease. However, with the hypnosis control of ANS dysfunction, it may only be an intellectual exercise as to the diagnosis, for hypnosis usually helps as it does in Raynaud's disease.

PRESSURE ON NERVES

Constant nerve impingement ranges from the ruptured disk syndromes to tumors that encroach on peripheral nerves and other sensitive tissues, such as the periosteum of bone or the capsule of an organ. Whether a tumor is growing in the bone and thereby causing expansion pain, or in the brain and causing constant headache due to expansion, or whether a tumor is impinging directly on a nerve trunk, there is a specific organic cause. This kind of pain, although chronic in the sense of time, can be understood best through the acute neurological model, and is therefore logical by any definition. Any ongoing pain, or other symptom, can be utilized by the human psyche as a way of dealing with life's problems, even though the pain was originally organic.

Hypnosis is usually not indicated for pain caused by a ruptured nucleus pulposus or slipped disk, at least until the diagnosis is determined. The patient's unconscious will prevent hypnosis control of the pain as a protection until the diagnosis is made. When it is safe to control the pain, hypnosis will then help.

There is a story, possibly apocryphal, that illustrates the *unconscious protection* inherent in hypnotherapy. A 40-year-old physician developed back and leg pain, which was not controlled by hypnosis. Soon, a diagnosis of a ruptured nucleus pulposus was made. Between the time that the definitive diagnosis was made and the successful surgery was performed, hypnosis and self-hypnosis controlled the pain. Several years later the pain returned, but this time the examining physician thought that the insurance coverage that benefited the patient during his previous illness had been so good he now was just wanting another "vacation." However, hypnosis did not control this pain. Several months later, a cancer involving the cauda equina in the lower part of the spine, was diagnosed. By then, it was too late to perform surgery; however, after the definitive cancer diagnosis was made, hypnosis gave him complete control of his pain and he died comfortably.

Hypnosis is often helpful in controlling pain caused by terminal cancer. The hypnosis maneuver, using the transfer of anesthesia from the hand where it has been hypnotically directed to the area of pain, is an ideal treatment in many cases and will often allow patients to dispense with narcotics and spend their last few weeks or months of life with a clear mind (Schafer 1984a,b). However, some terminal patients prefer to be in a narcotic fog. A successful case and one of a failure are presented to illustrate the complexity of these problems.

> A 50-year-old, married Caucasian woman was lying in her bed in the physical medicine and rehabilitation ward of the University of California, Irvine Medical Center with her right arm slightly elevated on a pillow. She had a pancoast tumor of the apex of the right lung, which had already extended from the apex into the large nerve trunks of the arm. Treatment had eventually resulted in the surgical transection all of the nerves involved in the brachial plexus above the point of the cancer, but with no relief of pain. Although she stated that her pain was severe and ongoing, she greeted me with a smile that seemed to belie her condition. She stated that she and her husband had an only daughter who was addicted to heroin and had married a heroin addict. In addition, she was not allowed to see her only granddaughter. Unconsciously, she felt her life was over, that it was her fault that she had failed their daughter

and that therefore she should die painfully as punishment. She did not go into hypnosis enough to gain any benefits, and died shortly thereafter.

A 42-year-old Caucasian man was in the terminal stages of carcinoma of the head of the pancreas. He was severely jaundiced and in such pain that high doses of morphine sulfate were giving minimal relief. I was constrained by his wife from telling him that he had cancer. I felt that he realized his diagnosis, but was "playing the game" expected of him, a phenomenon that I have observed frequently. I saw him alone, and found instant and excellent rapport. He went into hypnosis easily and was taught to anesthetize his hand and then transfer that lack of sensation to whatever area he desired relief. He never had another injection of morphine. His last two weeks of life were in the hospital after he developed gangrene of the feet. Although he was unable to reach these painful areas, I was able to instruct him on the telephone that a transfer of the anesthesia to the main nerves in his groin would do the same thing. His mind was clear until his terminal coma.

PERIPHERAL NEURITIS

The peripheral neuritic conditions are caused usually by diabetes, avitaminosis, chronic alcoholism, paresis, pernicious anemia, multiple sclerosis (although central in origin), and certain rare conditions. The overall treatment is specific to the disease. Many of the disease processes can be stopped, but in some cases the pain remains. These sufferers complain of a burning pain, which indicates an ANS origin. An exception to this is found in the thalamic syndrome, a painful condition caused by pathology in the thalamus. As explained in Chapter 6, hypnosis and self-hypnosis often offer control of ANS activity even in organic pathology, and is therefore important to consider in these patients for self-control. Guided imagery, usually via hypnosis, with feelings of standing in the cool surf offers symptomatic relief for many of these patients.

> A 75-year-old, Caucasian, retired college professor of philosophy was referred to me for hypnosis treatment of peripheral neuritis secondary to sarcoidosis. This autoimmune disease was also seen as the cause of his temporal arteritis, a rare complication of this condition. With hypnosis, he learned to imagine that he was standing in the cool surf. Following this, he soon experienced an ongoing relief of the painful burning sensation he had been complaining of. I also taught him to use overall muscle relaxation as a way of combatting stressors. He has had no recurrence of the pain or any of the symptoms of his primary illness, which was treated elsewhere before he had met me.

TRIGGER-POINT PAIN

Trigger points are discussed and illustrated in only a few textbooks and articles on pain (Travel and Simons

1983/1992). A trigger point is a point that, when irritated, produces pain in that area and/or at some distant point as well. These trigger points are palpably rather firm nodules or rope-like areas in the belly of a skeletal muscle that affects the striations of the muscles with added fat cells and mast cells. There is an accumulation of lactic acid in these nodules and muscles. When such a nodule or rope-like area is vigorously massaged, there is a jump or trigger response at the site or at the distant point of referred pain. Many times the injection of a local anesthetic, with or without one of the steroids, into a trigger point is the treatment of choice and will give instant and often permanent relief. Another treatment can be an ethyl chloride spray used cautiously so as not to freeze the skin. If not adequately treated, trigger points can result in "locked jaws," torticollis, and other difficulties. I am content to have these trigger-point pains, usually in the muscles or fascia, treated by injection until the injections are no longer needed. Interestingly enough, some of the most used acupuncture sites are at the places of the most frequently occurring trigger points. I have not found hypnotherapy to be of use in any of the trigger-point pains.

However, there are two specific pain syndromes that must be emphasized in the evaluation of the patient with the following unusually located trigger points.

Sphenopalatine Ganglian Neuralgia

This is a very painful headache, a hemicephalgia, which because of its rarity, leads the average physician into misdiagnosing the patient as a chronic hypochondriac. This headache occurs on only one-half of the head starting with the vertex and extending slightly lower into the upper cheek than would occur with a typical migraine headache. The patients complain in migraine-like terms that the pain is constant and not relieved by narcotics or tranquilizers. A pledget of cotton, on a small curved Kelly hemostat dipped in a solution of medical cocaine, when inserted into the nasopharynx and moved until the correct trigger area is found, will give instant and permanent relief.

Piriformis (Muscle) Syndrome

An involuntary spasm causes a painful cramping of the small piriformis muscle in the floor of the pelvis. This spasm of the muscle can be palpated by the gloved hand in either the vagina or the rectum. This muscle overlays the sciatic nerve as it enters the pelvis, and, if irritated by that spasm, gives a resulting spinal disk-like syndrome, which sometimes requires a spinal operation, obviously without relief. The proper treatment is the injection of a local anesthetic agent by a long needle guided by the gloved finger into the belly of the piriformis muscle, which gives instant and usually permanent relief (Figure 7–1).

POSTHERPETIC NEURALGIA

This very painful and debilitating condition, usually worse in the elderly, is caused by a virus, originally

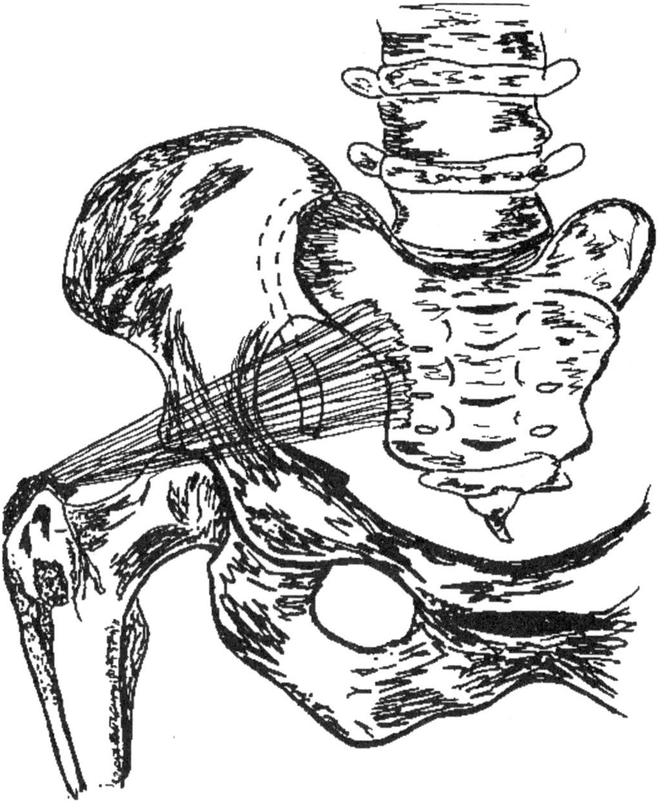

Figure 7–1.

PIRIFORMIS MUSCLE: runs from the side of the coccyx bone to the greater trochanter of the femur. Its purpose is to pull the leg outward and slightly rotate so that the involved foot has its toes over the other foot.

from childhood chickenpox. The pain is usually described as constant and intense with burning and other paresthesias. The syndrome starts with an attack of herpes zoster or shingles. The severe pain follows the affected peripheral nerve. It is thought that the acquired resistance to the chickenpox virus weakens over time, making it possible for shingles to occur. As scientifically unbelievable as it may seem, I have seen two cases where hypnosis relieved the pain while still in the prodromal period with only the initial redness present. Not only was the pain relieved by direct suggestion, but the lesions never formed. The lesions of this condition go through the chickenpox stages – macual, papual, vesicle, pustule – and finally a crust sloughs leaving a reddened partial pit, which usually fades without residuals, although sometimes pigmentation of a pit is present. It is probable that chickenpox can be transmitted from these lesions and the patient should be properly warned about contact with susceptible children. Most medical and many surgical treatments are not successful. However, hypnotherapy and teaching autohypnosis is the treatment of choice giving a high degree of success in a minimum of visits.

> An 80-year-old Caucasian man living in a retirement hotel with his wife was seen by me at the request of his internist because of overuse of percodan. His history revealed ten years of intense suffering in his right chest wall following an attack of shingles. The pain followed the route of the fourth intercostal nerve, which had been injected with Novocain, then alcohol, cut and finally subjected to a triple flap-raising operation. At the onset of his pain, he had become so depressed that a course of electroconvulsive treatments were given that relieved the depression but not the pain. I would have

diagnosed him as a career-pain patient but to my surprise, the first use of hypnosis resulted in an instant "cure," the only relief he had ever received. However, the pain returned the next day. The next visit resulted in the same temporary relief. On my third visit, I fortuitously found myself following him down the hall of the retirement hotel. With almost every step, he was stopped with questions from concerned friends as to his condition, to which he would answer with obvious signs of suffering. I realized that this pain identified him as an outstanding person in this hotel; but without it he would be just another old man. This time, I suggested while he was in hypnosis, that three or fewer Percodan would handle his pain adequately. He was able to accept this suggestion, which pleased all parties concerned.

THALAMIC SYNDROME

The thalamus is a group of nuclei in the middle of the brain (see Figure 3–1). It has many functions. All of the pain fibers make connections in one or more of these nuclei before being relayed further. Therefore, anything that would irritate any area of the thalamus would cause pain. The most common cause of thalamic pain is from strokes that occur near or in it. I shall report a rather unusual case, but one that does illustrate this condition.

A 19-year-old man from Yemen was referred to me from the neurosurgical department of the University of California, Irvine Medical Center. He was already diagnosed as having a *Schistosoma* (a small tropical worm) crawl into a blood vessel in his thalamus and die. This resulted in a right hemiparesis together with an intense burning sensation on the right side of his body. Although there was a language problem, I was able to successfully induce hypnosis and treat him, through an interpreter who spoke for me in Arabic, with suggestions for relief.

GOUT

Gout has been described through the ages (Hart 1983). Gout is an extremely painful condition that comes on suddenly, especially in the big toe (Alexander 1986). Its name comes from the Latin word *gutta,* meaning "drop," and was originally thought to be caused by drops of poison put into the joint by an angry goddess, Podagra, the food torturess (Cornelius and Schneider, 1988). Proper x-rays and needle aspirations of the involved joint may be necessary to confirm the diagnosis. Gout has a different origin than the other syndromes so far reported for it is a metabolic disease or condition. It is caused by high levels of uric acid in the bloodstream, which then precipitates out into crystals in the bones and joints as well as in some of the soft tissues of the body. When these crystals form in the "hard" tissues, pain results not just from the expansion of the tissues but also from irritation. Being a disease of metabolism, often with a hereditary origin, it offers certain measurements that should make it easy to diagnose; however, some early attacks are not diagnosed. When a blood chemistry profile is done, often routinely, the high uric acid level will confirm the diagnosis and distinguish it from trauma or another type of arthritis. It has a predilection for the large joint of the big toe, a significant sign in any adult male of any age or female over 45. However, it can occur in any joint. If it occurs in the temperomandibular joint, it is usually not recognized as gout even if that diagnosis has been made about other areas of the body.

The treatment of gout is relatively simple, for it first consists of dietarily lowering the purines found especially in meat and seafoods. Also certain medications lower the blood uric acid level. However, dieting should be undertaken carefully, for a change in metabolism can precipitate the uric acid crystals, as may the intake of diuretics. The nonsteroidal anti-inflammatory drugs (NSAIDs) are excellent for reversing the inflammation and therefore the pain. In the more severe conditions involving gout, a rheumatologist may be consulted.

SICKLE CELL ANEMIA

This genetic condition of African-Americans, involving misshapen red blood cells that can get caught in the smaller arterioles of large parts of the body, causes terrible pain when an attack occurs. It is felt that many attacks occur at times of stress. Hypnotherapy will help these patients control much of their stress. Also, especially during an attack, direct suggestion during hypnosis with appropriate posthypnotic suggestions and instructions in self-hypnosis will help these patients deal with pain without resorting to narcotics.

COSTOCHONDRITIS

This not too rare a condition, formerly known as Costen's syndrome as well as Tietze's syndrome, is mentioned, not because it is difficult to diagnose, but because it sends the patient into a panic, since it is experienced as a possible heart attack. Whenever a person gets a pain in the chest, it is considered to originate in the heart until proven otherwise. It is therefore good judgment to be taken to the emergency room to be sure of the diagnosis. After the usual examination, including a physical examination, electrocardiograms, blood assays, and others, a clean bill of health for the heart is acknowledged and the diagnosis of costochondritis is made. This condition sometimes follows physical activity, but many times has no cause. Some see it also as a stress disease. Very simply, it is an irritation on either or both sides of the sternum where the cartilage meets the bone of the affected ribs. The experience of this pain, especially when on the left side, is the cause of the patient's distressed feelings. Restricted activity as well as the anti-inflammatory medications will help until healing takes place.

Because some of these syndromes are rare enough that they are not recognized by many physicians, it might be necessary for a patient to find proper treatment by calling a number of doctors to see if they are familiar with the disorder. There are many well-read patients who may try self-diagnosis, and thereby put physicians "on the spot." If it is in one of the syndromes that I have identified as often responding to hypnosis, it may be necessary to find a physician who is familiar with the disorder and who either utilizes hypnosis or can cooperate with a health professional who does. A description and discussion of these conditions will enable health professionals to make better diagnoses.

8

SPECIFIC PAIN SYNDROMES DIFFICULT TO DIAGNOSE

This chapter discusses pain problems that are often unrecognized and misunderstood by doctors.

FACET STRAIN

This condition is often overlooked as just another low back syndrome. However, it can be treated in most cases if it is recognized and diagnosed properly. The patient complains of low back pain that occurs in the middle of the night but not during the day. Usually, the patient states that getting up and having a glass of milk or walking around the house for ten to twenty minutes results in the pain going away, at which time the patient returns to bed and finishes a night of otherwise good sleep.

Each vertebra rests its two lower facets on the top two of the next vertebra. These are the supporting structures of the spinal column, for the disk between the vertebrae is a cushion rather than a support. Each facet joint, where the upper and lower ones come together, is "wrapped" in various ligaments to hold it solidly in place. When one sleeps in such a position that these ligaments are strained, this back pain will occur. Walking relieves the strain placed on the ligaments by the sleep position and the pain goes away. A few strengthening exercises and a mild readjustment of the sleeping position will usually give relief. However, it is almost impossible to change habitual sleeping positions, so the aim should be to reposition a knee or an arm slightly, keeping the mechanics of the back in mind. Occasionally, this conservative approach will not work, and injection of a local anesthetic with some steroid into these small joints will be necessary. Hypnotherapy does not result in relief, for this pain is an acute one that signals the patient that something is wrong and that s/he must readjust the back in some manner. As emphasized previously, "failures" in hypnosis can be very diagnostic (Schafer 1989) and should alert the physician to reconsider the situation. This condition must be differentiated from spondylolisthesis, which is a congenitally slanted facet condition causing facet strain in the upright position and is correctable through surgery.

A 56-year-old woman came to me with the complaint of severe neck pain resulting from an automobile accident followed by surgery, five years previously. She informed me that if she was very careful and performed little work, her neck pain was not too severe; however, since she must work for a living, longer work hours caused a great deal of suffering, especially in the evenings. Hypnosis and self-hypnosis gave her almost immediate control of this pain, but she informed me that it did not help her low back pain during the night, which she had not previously described. Further investigation of this pain revealed a typical facet strain condition. When it was explained that simple suppression of the pain was contraindicated, for it was a signal that something was wrong and required attention, she accepted walking for fifteen minutes in the middle of the night for relief. She was also helped with exercise to strengthen the involved muscles and to shift her sleeping position slightly.

OSTEOARTHRITIS

This type of arthritis entails the acute recurrent pain of the psychosomatic syndromes, but its cause is often not recognized; when it is, the patient can often be treated and receive complete relief. Although osteoarthritis is a condition of aging and of wear and tear, it is not a universal one. Some individuals who lead very physical lives are not afflicted, whereas some who do little physical work suffer severe cases in early middle age. The stresses and strains of living are reflected in the muscle tensions of these patients, for it is the mild but steady minimal muscle tension that causes the bony pathology. The origins and insertions of muscles near the joints experience this mild and almost constant strain. The resultant irritation of the bone and cartilage at the affected areas leads to inflammations, pain, and deformity, often with resulting bone spurs (Figure 8–1).

Psychotherapy may uncover the reasons for this patient's mild, ongoing muscle tension. Teaching the patient to relax, especially if enhanced with hypnosis and self-hypnosis will give relief, whether or not blood chemistry changes have been noted. It is likely that these chemical changes are a result of the inflammatory process, not the other way around. There are many treatments for this condition, including aspirin, non-steroidal anti-inflammatory drugs (NSAIDs), calcium, hormones, heat and cold, and exercises.

> A 60-year-old woman had such severe osteoarthritis that she was unable to walk for more than twenty minutes. After examining the stresses in her life, I was able not only to help her deal with them better, but I taught her self-hypnosis and bodily relaxation. She is now able to walk and even go dancing.

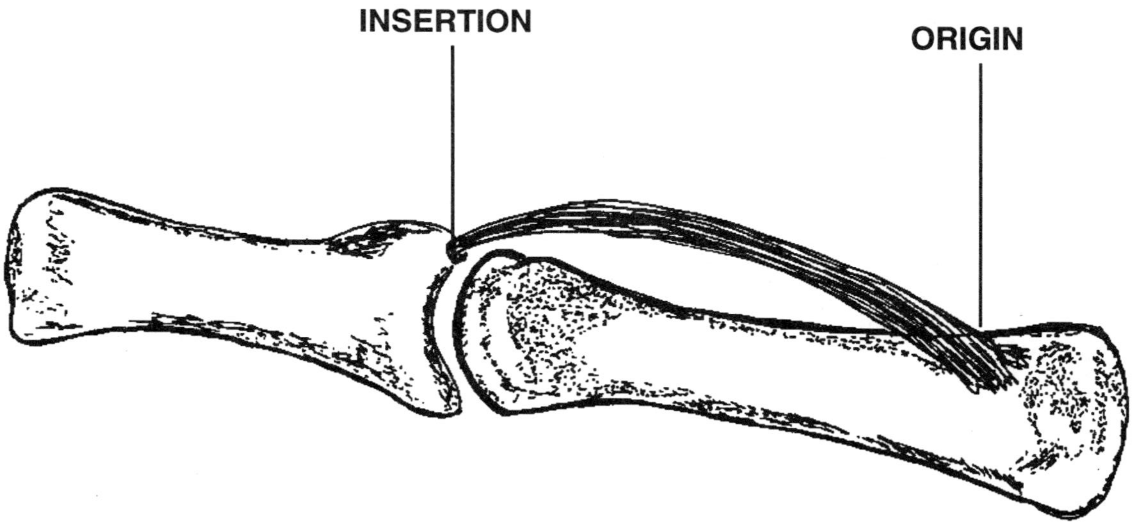

Figure 8–1.

OSTEOARTHRITIS: When this hypothetical muscle joint is almost continually in mild tension, it causes irritation at the sight of insertion, near the joint. It also tends to pull out a spur of bone. The irritation causes an inflammatory reaction which is then reflected in the changes in the chemistry in the blood stream, which is measurable in the tests for arthritis.

PALINDROMIC RHEUMATISM

The name of this condition is misleading, for it is not a "rheumatism" but rather a rare condition not easily recognized and diagnosed. It is also probably one of the psychosomatic conditions, for it is an acute recurrent illness and stress related. It is a fleeting polyarthritis that attacks mostly the smaller joints, especially of the hands and feet. The pain is almost unbearable, lasts only a few days, and is usually relieved by an NSAID. It may move on to another joint or leave if the "attack" is over, only to return at the next bout of stress. Meningococcal and gonococcal arthritis as well as rheumatic fever must be ruled out.

ARACHNOIDITIS

The thickening of the arachnoid membrane of the spinal cord can occur from injury, infection, and other conditions, but much of this thickening is caused by the irritation of x-ray contrast media in myelographic studies. In recent years, most of these studies are now being done noninvasively by positron emission tomography (PET) scans, computed tomography (CT) scans, and magnetic resonance imaging (MRI). One or even two of the contrast media studies would usually do no harm, but more would be asking for trouble. When the membrane is irritated it thickens, and the nerves are mildly irritated at the point they leave the canal, leading to patchy areas of altered sensation – hypoesthesia, hyperesthesia, paresthesia, and anesthesia. In many cases, hypnotherapy gives at least some self-control and relief from the discomfort, especially if the patient comprehends the condition.

> A 47-year-old Caucasian woman had sustained a low back injury in an automobile accident seven years previous to seeing me. She had undergone stabilizing surgery, but complained of severe low back pain. Four contrast media studies by four different specialists did not reveal further disk damage. By the time I saw her in my office, she had patches, from her hips down, of numbness, pain, prickling sensations, and some varying feelings of heat and cold. Hypnotherapy in five hourly sessions taught her self-hypnosis with visualizations of healing and normalizing the blood flow and nerve impulses. This gave her the ability to control the pain and ignore the other different feelings as long as she restricted her physical activities. With this control, she was able to live a relatively comfortable life. In my experience, the presence of ongoing litigation usually precludes such good results.

MULTIPLE PERSONALITY DISORDER

This complex syndrome is discussed in detail elsewhere (Schafer 1986). These patients have unusual ways of handling their pain. Many times this comes up in therapy and in the history, and can contribute to making the diagnosis of the syndrome.

When abreacting and living through a previous abusive incident, patients will have not only the pain of that incident return, but also other physical signs. I treated one patient who had what appeared to be finger marks around her neck during a session in which she was describing the pain of being almost strangled by her mother at the age of 5 or 6. Another patient had a somewhat similar set of symptoms accompanying the return of memories of her mother's boyfriend attempting to hang her with a rope.

The reverse can also happen. Another patient told me of her abusive ex-husband having bent back her little finger and breaking it during an argument. She stated that she had no feeling of pain when this happened. It seems that one of her alter personalities, who came into existence during childhood to handle pain, had taken over so that her main personality did not feel anything.

Hypnosis is often not necessary in the diagnosis and treatment of this condition because the patients may intuitively, although unconsciously, place themselves in what we observe to be self-hypnosis in order to access an alter personality. As a defense, they dissociate into *another personality*. This was a survival tool at the time of the original abuse.

SPASMODIC TORTICOLLIS

This is a frequently seen syndrome that is easily diagnosed. However, physical treatment rarely works and the surgical treatment is almost barbaric. Hypnotherapy is not always successful, but understanding this condition is possible through a study of the patient's psyche, which is causing the soma to react with a *wry neck*. The alternative injection of botulinum toxin is also unnecessary in most circumstances. The physical culprit in this condition is the opposite-sided sternocleidomastoid muscle, which is spastically pushing the head in the opposite direction. This should be the therapeutic tipoff as to the origin. The therapist must explore the patient's background to find why s/he must turn the head (eyes) from something that is probably now symbolic of a previous traumatic occurrence.

> A 49-year-old Caucasian woman was married to an obese man who was somewhat older and whose health was failing. With his first symptoms of ill health, she developed her wry neck. Exploration of her background revealed that when she was 15 to 18 years old, she had to care for her father during his last illness caused by a stroke. She said that her father was quite prudish so that when she had to bathe him, she would avert her eyes from his genital area as well as from his rectal area. Her gaining this insight let her understand what it was that she would have to see when her husband became bedridden. Her head then straightened.

Complete investigation of this condition is necessary, especially physically, because a few organic causes can result in this syndrome. Also, if the head and neck have been held tightly in this position, certain resulting physical changes could occur that would prevent true correction even if psychologically cured. The cutting of part of the involved muscle is not reversible; psychotherapy, with or without hypnotherapy, should be utilized before any destructive surgery is considered.

WHOLE BODY PAIN

Some individuals who have suffered serious physical trauma experience upon awakening a feeling of pain that "proves I am still alive." This pain, which is a signal of ongoing life, is retained as if the loss of the pain would mean death. Ewin (1980) feels that if the injury is preceded by an emotional spurt of adrenaline at the time of the trauma, this whole body pain is most likely to result. He has done experimental animal studies that strongly support the validity of this concept. Hypnotherapy involves asking the patient to tentatively relinquish the pain for gradually progressive time periods with the "discovery" that s/he can indeed live without that pain.

9

HEADACHE

Evidence of trephination found in primitive graves and in the more advanced ancient civilizations indicate that headaches have always been with us. The early headache may have been seen as an internal and infernal demon, or as a result of an injury, or almost anything reflected in that culture. Today our knowledge of the causes of headaches is still far from complete.

A systematic approach is necessary in evaluating someone who is suffering from such an affliction. The physician needs to know the when, where, and how in order to find out the what. However, not enough doctors are trained to investigate why? Until the reason for the headache is established, treatment can be only symptomatic.

For good diagnostic evaluation, we need to know more about the pain: its frequency and time of day; sharpness or dullness; where it starts and where it extends; whether it affects any of the sense organs or muscular groups; whether someone else in the family or a close friend had or now has such a condition; whether it is accompanied by dizziness, lachrymation, salivation, or perspiration; and if anything seems to help or make it worse. Results of previous examinations and treatments are important so as to prevent repeating expensive procedures, such as CT, PET, and MRI, unless indicated. If these scans are used, hypnosis can help the patient cope better with the claustrophobic feelings engendered by these examinations. These scans eliminate the need for repeated spinal taps and spinal diagnostic injections. Psychotherapists should not make a diagnosis of emotional etiology on the basis of negative findings on the scans. Cooperation among the various diagnostic specialists is essential in arriving at a diagnosis. The assumption that everything is biological and must be treated physically and chemically is probably responsible for many of the failures in the treatment of headaches.

The indication for psychotherapy and especially hypnotherapy has been ignored because of a belief by many physicians that any result from such treatment is bogus, or at best temporary. (There is an anecdote about an old farmer who sees a giraffe and mutters as he walks away, "There is no such animal.") The modern psychiatric emphasis on biology is, in my estimation, interfering with the proper diagnosis and treatment of many headache sufferers. A biological understanding and treatment is important but symptomatic treatment is not enough when a permanent cure is a possibility.

Headaches can be classified as extracranial, intracranial, and functional or psychosomatic. The physical and the functional aspects are equally important, whether or not the physical origin is intracranial. This is especially true with vascular headaches, where the symptoms are temporary, recurrent, and usually responsive to psychotherapy with hypnotherapy.

EXTRACRANIAL HEADACHES

Sinusitis

Acute sinusitis is usually not difficult to diagnose. Since it is an infection of a sinus or sinuses, there are signs and symptoms of infection, often with fever and toxicity. There are four sinus areas: the bilateral frontals and maxillaries, and the deeper ethmoids and sphenoids. The pains from the acutely infected sinuses are caused by occlusion of the openings from the mucous membrane–lined pockets in the large bones of the face. The pressure within the sinus builds up and is responsible for the pain. If the infections are restricted to the ethmoids and the sphenoids, the diagnosis may be more difficult. Often an immediately preceding cold, flu, or allergic reaction helps point to the diagnosis. Antibiotics are usually administered effectively in those cases with a bacterial infection. However, if the condition becomes chronic, it is more difficult to diagnose and treat. Not too long ago, operative procedures were utilized, often as a last resort. However, this is seldom needed in our modern era because of antibiotics, antiallergy medications, and the agents that shrink the mucous membranes. Both acute and chronic sinusitis are less common now than before 1950. Except for the emotional involvement often seen in the allergies, treatment is usually biological. The allergies can be approached through hypnotherapy, for the autonomic nervous system, although thought to be autonomous, is really very close to conscious control, especially in the trance state during hypnotherapy. I recommend the visualization method. (See Chapter 4 for the maneuver I call the magic journey.)

PERIPHERAL NERVE PATHOLOGY

Any pathology involving the peripheral nerves of the head, neck, face, and mouth may present with symptoms of some kind of headache. The most significant ones are trigeminal neuralgia (tic douloureaux), herpes zoster, and sphenopalatine ganglion syndrome. Temporal arteritis is probably primarily an inflammatory process of the arteries, an autoimmune condition. Sphenopalatine ganglion neuralgia is discussed in Chapter 6.

Trigeminal Neuralgia (Tic Douloureux)

This is a poorly understood affliction of the third division of the fifth cranial nerve in which sudden excruciating pain affects that side of the face. This pain is lance-like, sudden, and intense. It tends to occur in the elderly, but is not exclusive to that age group. The pain occurs at unpredictable times, although almost any touch will set it off. Complete immobilization does not stop the paroxysms. Various injections and surgical excisions have been used in the past and refined now so that the frequent and terrible resulting numbness is not extensive. Nevertheless, many patients feel that this numbness is worse than the original pain.

In my observation, the elderly person with this condition is usually depressed. The depression may be involved in the etiology rather than resulting from the pain. Since it would seem that anyone with this condition would be depressed, most victims are not treated for the depression as such. One of the first things a physician should do is to consider prescribing an antidepressant. Since the pain attack seems almost epileptoid, some of the medications associated with seizure disorders have occasionally helped, and should be tried, for example, phenytoin (usually called Dilantin), carbamazepine, and baclofen. But most important is a thorough psychiatric history to determine if the patient is somaticizing some conflict.

A 56-year-old, Caucasian, married scientist was prescribed Tegretol, which had helped him for about two weeks, after which his symptoms returned in all of their intensity. He was then referred to me by his neurologist to see if hypnosis would give him any relief. It did not. The history revealed that his father, an engineer, had immigrated to the United States in 1914, leaving his family in Australia for a year, at which time he sent for them. On arrival, mother determined that the father had been having a torrid affair with another woman. After much stressful arguing, the parents decided to continue the marriage for the sake of the family, including this patient who was 10 years old at the time.

In adult life after he was married, my patient informed me that his wife had always been "cold," and that their adult children had understood and even encouraged him to divorce her and marry his recently widowed secretary. He said that she was everything that his wife was not. In addition, his wife had a good job, and the split of community property would leave her in a good financial position. I asked him if his mother ever impulsively slapped him in anger on the left cheek when he was a child, since the tic was on his left side. He answered in the affirmative. We worked with the following dynamics: He was repeating what his father had done, and his (internalized) mother was slapping him in the face because he was handling the situation differently. Within the next six sessions, his tic faded and he was well. I saw him about five years later and he informed me that he had indeed married his secretary and that they were living happily. His tic did not return.

There is very little in the hypnosis literature about this condition. Shafer (1962) described two cases treated quite permissively by teaching autohypnosis: self-anesthesia of an index finger and using that finger as a syringe to inject Novocain into the affected part. He accomplished complete and permanent cure of his two patients. Milne (1995) relates the case of a young woman whose attack periods were associated with stress. Hypnotherapy gave her control of her symptomatology for long periods of time. There are other paroxysmal neuralgias, both in the head area and in other parts of the body, but this is the most frequently seen.

Herpes Zoster

This very painful condition often called shingles follows the affected nerve root and is probably caused by the chickenpox virus, as explained in Chapter 6. This illness is especially serious if the nerve that runs over the cornea is involved, for it can lead to permanent opacity of the cornea with blindness. Hypnotherapy is of exceptional value, as discussed in Chapter 6, in possibly aborting the condition, if recognized early enough, or at least in making the patient more comfortable. It is very helpful in the postherpetic pain syndrome. Although there are some medications that now seem to alleviate at least some of the pain, I feel that hypnotherapy is the approach of choice because it gives the patient control of this symptom without adding more medications. And if it does not work, the therapist can explore the secondary gains that would often defeat a pharmacological approach.

Temporal Arteritis

This is not primarily a peripheral nerve problem, but one of inflammation of the arteries. Especially in older adults, quick medical attention is indicated for it can lead to stroke or blindness. Often, there is low-grade fever, vision difficulties, weight loss, and pain on one side while chewing, which sometimes leads to a wrong diagnosis of temporomandibular joint dysfunction. Often accompanying the headache is a burning pain around the ear where the temporal artery is inflamed. Treatment usually includes high doses of corticosteroids as well as other anti-inflammatory agents.

Temporomandibular Joint (TMJ) Syndrome

Although dental conditions can present as headaches, we will concentrate on the area of the head that seems to be most puzzling to both dentists and physicians. This disorder, which is a combination of muscle spasm and destructive lesions of the joint, probably as a result of that spasm, is usually treated mechanically with bite preventers, and raising or lowering the teeth. The pain of the TMJ is often thought to be migraine by many patients and some physicians, for it is often only on one side of the head and tends to fan out higher on the face and head to the temporal and parietal areas. Naturally, migraine medication does not give relief. Trigger-point lesions in the area muscles must also be ruled out. The injection of a local anesthetic agent into the trigger point will be diagnostic and sometimes curative. To complicate the matter, migraine, TMJ, and trigger-point pain can occur at the same time, confusing the diagnosis and treatment.

It is my opinion that the TMJ syndrome is psychosomatic. The teeth are the first organs of aggression, for the child learns to bite early in life, and many of these patients are unconsciously somaticizing their anger by clamping and/or gritting and grinding their teeth. A further problem is that the involved muscles can be in spasm without the usual continuing symptoms of clenching or bruxing. Yoga demonstrates that control of muscles and muscle groups can be trained consciously. The unconscious can do the same thing both here and, as we will see later, in the neck muscles in tension headaches. The following case history illustrates the interplay between the psyche and the soma, whereas an earlier, purely mechanical, approach had failed.

> A 37-year-old, native Korean woman the mother of four, married to an American blue collar worker, was seen in the Hypnotherapy and Pain Evaluation Center by a social worker. Her complaint was of severe left TMJ pain of ten years' duration during which time her teeth had been built

> up, ground down, and then removed, so that all the upper and lower teeth from the midline on the left side had been pulled. Her history revealed that she was born in Korea, was prostituted by her older brother from an early age so that the family could subsist. She then married an American enlisted man and had two children by him before being divorced when he returned to the States. After being further prostituted by her brother, she married another G.I., and after two more children, came to the States with him at the end of his tour of duty. They had a good marriage and family life until her guilt feelings about her family had her send for them. As they arrived, her TMJ pain began, followed by her odyssey through the dental offices. After we received this information, we "taught" her that her first responsibilities were toward her marriage and children, not primarily to her family of origin. Additionally, she gained insight into her forbidden anger at her family. She was also taught self-hypnosis for the control of pain. In five hourly visits, her symptoms disappeared. At a follow-up five months later, there had been no return of symptoms.

This discussion is not meant to criticize those who practice dentistry; rather it is to suggest that the purely mechanical approach to TMJ patients is not sufficient. Those who do not respond readily must be investigated for unconscious ongoing psychosomatic problems that might be amenable to psychotherapy and particularly hypnotherapy. Most symptoms happen for a reason that is not necessarily organic.

Other dental problems must also be considered when investigating headache. An abscessed tooth, especially in the upper back area of the jaw, can cause referred pain into the ear as well as into the temporal area. An abscess that extends into the maxillary sinus can also cause headaches.

Cervical Area Pathology

Muscular imbalance, strains such as those associated with whiplash injuries, disk disease of the cervical spine, cervical arthritis, spasmodic torticollis, and other conditions involving the neck are mentioned here as possible sources of headache. The mastoid area must also be examined, especially if there is a history of middle ear infection, although this condition has become relatively rare with antibiotics. The lymph glands can also be a cause of headaches, as can some lymphomas. Primary as well as metastatic carcinoma must also be considered, as rare as this may be, for it can involve areas in the head as well as in the extracranial areas.

Eye and Eye Muscle Pathology

This group of conditions requires a good eye examination to make the differential diagnosis of headache, but this is outside the scope of this chapter.

Acute Recurrent Tension Headache

This headache originates in the back of the neck and involves the paraspinal neck muscles. They extend into the muscles of the back of the head as well as over the scalp. Many people experience this condition as originating in the frontal sinuses (which may themselves be inflamed). However, this is primarily a psychosomatic condition with a typical "body language" communicative aspect (see Chapter 5). I always look for the "pain in the neck" in the patient's life. Psychotherapy including hypnotherapy will help this patient tremendously. If the condition is of long standing, the migraine maneuver (Chapter 4) often works.

Scalp Muscle Contraction Headache

This relatively rare condition is experienced as a feeling of crawling and wriggling of the scalp muscles. Many of these patients fear that they are going crazy. This is a special type of tension headache with its origins in stress and anxiety. It is listed in *Classification of Chronic Pain* (Merskey and Bogduk 1994) as a chronic condition, but I feel it is more easily understood as an acute recurrent pain, and therefore a psychosomatic condition. During attacks, it is felt as a dull aching head pain and is often generalized. Hypnosis helps and gives the patient better control. Biofeedback is also an excellent treatment, but usually is used empirically without attempts to understand the dynamics.

A 65-year-old African-American woman, retired as a school administrator, was married to a black foreign-born physician, who spent more time and interest on his patients and co-workers than on his wife who had put him through medical school. The scalp contractions started when she realized that her husband had used her more for his education than out of affection. When she first saw me, she was obsessed with the feeling that this symptom was proof that she was going crazy. After getting to know her in about ten visits, I suddenly looked at her and suggested emphatically that if she was going to go crazy she should do it now when I could see that she was taken to the right hospital. When she realized that I was quite serious, she finally accepted that she was not going crazy, and we were able to progress in therapy. She was moderately good at visualizing a comfortable haven. This gave her the ability to alleviate her symptoms somewhat, and to give her attention to other areas of her life and cope much better. Although her symptoms did not disappear, she has done very well. She uses her symptoms now as a way of evaluating areas of tension in her life. She is also helped by 50 mg of Elavil and two 2 mg of Valium a day.

Caffeine Withdrawal Headache

Withdrawal from any substance can be associated with headache. But the caffeine withdrawal headache can be one of the most puzzling conditions seen in headache clinics because most patients do not associate coffee with anything "bad." This should be easily diagnosed, but most patients do not volunteer that they drink coffee, let alone that it could be the cause. It is very difficult to get these patients to slowly eliminate this substance from their daily life. An acquired sensitivity does not seem logical to them. Treating headache with minor narcotics, regardless of the origins of that headache, many times sets up a vicious cycle with the unconscious fear of the headache preventing the withdrawal of the medication. The cycle follows when the fear of being without the medication unconsciously causes the headache. This is often complicated because withdrawal from a substance, coffee as well as medications like codeine, may be the cause of the ongoing headache syndrome.

Substance Withdrawal Headache

When substances are used for treatment of any syndrome, the patient can become habituated if not actually addicted. Many chronic, career-pain patients are hooked on the minor narcotics or the tranquilizers. This is especially true of many chronic and chronic recurrent headaches. Attempts to try new medications and to readjust those already being used usually ends in failure. Withdrawal of these substances is necessary for definitive treatment of many conditions where it is obvious to the treating physician that they are doing no good. The symptoms persist in a vicious manner on even the threat of very slow withdrawal. Many times hospitalization is necessary to effect this withdrawal.

The following is the case of a headache patient, already registered as an addict, whom I was able to challenge in such a way that I successfully treated her as an outpatient. (Some state laws forbid treating such patients as outpatients if they are in any way addicted to any of the narcotics, minor or major [Joranson 1995].)

> I treated a 45-year-old housewife with a complaint of severe generalized headaches of ten years' duration. Each day she was taking between 35 and 40 aspirin preparations with one grain of codeine in each tablet. She realized that she was addicted, and had been registered as an addict by her primary physician, who was at his wit's end with her. Her headache had started when she was under a great deal of domestic strain from both sets of parents moving into her home. Additionally, two of her four children had congenital defects that caused concern and required much attention. I explained to her that I had never been able to help a person eliminate that much medication without hospitalization. When she refused to be institutionalized, I challenged her with a routine of eliminating one daily tablet each week, meanwhile giving her a great deal of ego support, practical advice about her daily life, and hypnotherapy to teach her to relax. To my surprise, she was able to follow this routine, and eliminated the last three of her daily pills as a

New Year's resolution. Her next two weeks were the first time she was without headache. After a few more sessions, she saw herself as cured and vowed never to take another narcotic.

INTRACRANIAL HEADACHES

Expanding Lesions

However obvious these conditions appear to be, they are often not diagnosed when they should have been. A complete physical examination, including a neurological examination with emphasis on the reflexes and an ophthalmoscopic examination, is indicated in all conditions of headache. Many primary or secondary cancers and brain abscesses will be uncovered, as well as some aneurysms and hematomas. The eye grounds may reveal other conditions as well. Intracranial hemorrhages and thromboses will make their presence known in other ways. There are many diagnostic procedures that can then be relied upon to finalize the diagnosis.

Any infectious process involving the meninges will be manifested by headache. Bacterial and virus invasion, parasites, and toxins such as carbon monoxide and lead must be considered. An injury must never be ignored, for a slowly bleeding subdural hematoma is life threatening and can result from what seems to be a minor injury several days or even weeks previously.

With the widespread use of blood thinners, this hematoma, though rare, can even occur spontaneously.

Postmeningitis Syndrome

This is an ill-defined headache syndrome that is sometimes seen following meningitis. Also, headaches often accompany incidents of severe stress, with or without head trauma. Many of these headaches are of neurotic origin and might now be seen as part of a posttraumatic stress disorder. Each may be further complicated by damage to the cerebral tissue itself with acute or chronic brain conditions.

Hydrocephalis

This must be considered for it is not always restricted to children or to people from the tropics infested with parasites, malarial or otherwise. Proper treatment of the primary condition is obvious. Neurosurgical intervention is sometimes required.

Post–Spinal Tap Headache

This headache occurs following a tap into the spinal canal for either an examination or a spinal anesthetic. If the needle hole does not "plug up" spontaneously, fluid will continue to drip slowly into the tissues. If the amount of fluid lost in this way is excessive, the brain will, in a manner of speaking, rattle around in the skull, causing the headache with any movement. This is a purely mechanical phenomenon, and almost always clears up in a few days. Quietly lying flat in bed is the usual remedy.

HEADACHES OF PSYCHOSOMATIC ORIGIN

Headaches that afflict almost everyone from time to time, especially when we are upset or annoyed, whether we want to admit it to ourselves or not, are probably vascular and spastic in origin and are relieved by aspirin or Tylenol (acetaminophen). The newer group of medications called antiprostaglandins (one of the group of medicines referred to as NSAIDs) are more frequently being used as over-the-counter medications. Physicians should urge their patients to stay with the tried and true, aspirin and Tylenol, as long as they relieve the symptoms. Any headache that does not respond, and for which a cause isn't obvious, calls for a thorough medical examination.

Migraine

Although most people call any severe headache migraine, a classic migraine is characterized by severe pain involving one side and a preceding aura of some unusual feeling in the head, face, or even stomach. Scintillating scotomata, nausea, and vomiting, and occasionally central neurological signs, also occur. Migraine variants include histamine headaches, cluster headaches, and allergic ones. Cluster headaches cluster in time, not anatomically. I prefer to deal with all of these as one condition as well as any one-sided headache other than the sphenopalatine ganglian syndrome headache (Chapter 6).

> The wife of a patient I had previously treated sought my help for her headaches that started around the end of November and ended the next Easter. Her history revealed that she was the second born in a Jewish family with an older favorite brother who was allowed to express his sibling rivalry extensively; however, my patient was not allowed to reciprocate. Her first therapy appointment after the New Year revealed a severe migraine at one minute past midnight. With some further inquiry, it was possible to interpret that the symbol for the New Year was the birth of a baby boy, which followed the season celebrating the birth of Jesus, a first-born Jewish baby boy. After working through these ideas, and the parallels to her family situation, her headaches never returned.

The pathophysiological problem in migraine consists primarily of spasm of the smooth muscles in the walls of the involved intracranial arteries, especially in the extra- or subdural area, which causes most of what are referred to as the migraine prodromal symptoms such as the aura and scintillating scotomata. It is then followed by dilatation of the blood vessels accompanied by edema of their walls, which account for most of the pain since bone does not allow for expansion.

The routine treatment involves medications such as ergot preparations and beta blockers. These medications must be given early or prophylactically to relieve or prevent the initial spasm of an attack. This is really only symptomatic treatment, and does not influence the condition itself. Histamine desensitization may help, but I am not sure that this "cure" isn't a deconditioning of the symptoms rather than a desensitization to histamine. I see migraine as a dysfunction of the involved autonomic nervous system caused by intrapsychic conflicts. This is especially true early in the course of the illness. Therefore, migraine headaches must be treated psychotherapeutically to effect a cure, otherwise the usual medicinal approach is only palliative. Hypnotherapy is ideal, especially as a short-term therapeutic approach, and will usually uncover the antecedents involved in the condition. Although there is often a parent with the same complaint, in my opinion this does not mean migraines are genetic. The process of identifying with the other afflicted person often explains the migraines of a patient.

The concept of a psychosomatic symptom becoming simply a conditioned response has not been well examined. As background, Pavlov's dog salivated at the sight of meat, then salivated at the sight of meat and the ringing of a bell, finally it salivated with just the ringing of the bell. In some complicated manner, many migraines, as well as other conditions, continue to occur from such conditioning after the early era of the attacks (see Chapter 5). If such a patient is seen in my office in the first three years of his/her migraines, I will probably have to "therapeutize" that patient, for simple hypnosis will usually not influence the headache even if a "failure" helps make the diagnosis. However, I welcome seeing a patient who has had migraines for ten or more years. The following example illustrates this.

> A 75-year-old Caucasian widow gave a history of severe migraine of 54 years' duration. For the last several months she had been treated in the hospital emergency room almost weekly for severe attacks needing intermuscular Demerol in 75- to 100-mg amounts. After taking her history, I induced a hypnotic trance and taught her the migraine maneuver (Chapter 4). She has been free of headaches for over three years at this writing.

It is probable that the treatment of cluster headache must include a period during which the attack is going on. Each cluster headache patient has his/her own pattern, and usually erroneous ideas as to the cause. The treatment, otherwise, is the same as with the migraine maneuver.

By categorizing headaches into three groups, extracranial, intracranial, and psychosomatic, I have emphasized the differential diagnoses of many conditions. I have also described where and how hypnotherapy is indicated. The case histories illustrate where hypnotherapy is the tool of choice, and some cases where it is not. It is especially valuable in treating migraine headaches and tension neck/headache. Both of these conditions are discussed in detail in Chapter 5.

10

PAIN AS A PRESENTING SYMPTOM OF PSYCHIATRIC CONDITIONS

Often pain is purely of psychological origin; additionally, disorders of the mind can present themselves as pain. The manner in which this happens cannot easily be explained but is briefly addressed in Chapter 3. As further clarification, we must always remember that all psychological symptoms are unconscious defenses of the ego even if they are not very logical in the patient's world. This is especially true when depression is experienced as a somatic symptom; we then refer to the symptom as a *depressive equivalent.* Pain can also be a *schizophrenic equivalent,* but is rarely recognized as such. We also have *neurotic equivalents,* which are referred to by other terms such as *conversion symptoms* and *somatoform pain disorders,* as it is called in the *Diagnostic and*

Statistical Manual (*DSM-IV*) (American Psychiatric Association 1994). Furthermore, the manual differentiates these two terms, for the conversion diagnosis does not include pain as a prominent part of the condition. Also, pain as a somatic memory is not discussed in *DSM-IV*, or in any other book of which I am aware. This chapter discusses it. A final category is "iatrogenic."

Other than the somatoform disorders, the conditions referred to in this chapter are not covered in *DSM-IV*. They are holdovers from earlier *DSM* editions. Many of the following conditions must therefore be viewed as unofficial names of psychiatric illnesses.

DEPRESSIVE EQUIVALENTS

Although depression is considered an important part of most patients' reactions to pain, especially in the chronic conditions, pain is also at least a partial way of handling the depression, not necessarily the cause of it. Many treatment approaches to the chronic pain patient include the use of antidepressant medication, even though many physicians only visualize the nerve pathways that might be involved, seeing the depression as caused by the pain. This kind of thinking should be reversed, for the pain only disguises the depression as much as it can; the patient is primarily depressed. There are other equivalents associated with depression. For example, pathological obesity can be a depressive equivalent and sometimes a schizophrenic equivalent.

Hypochondria is also a depressive equivalent, but has so many other aspects that we would be going far afield if we tried to examine that condition here.

As in any of the equivalent conditions, the first suspicion arises when no objective signs are found to account for the pain. Trying an antidepressant at this time is definitely indicated, even if prescribed eclectically. If it fails, and there is still no reason to believe that an organic condition exists, electroconvulsive treatment should be considered. This almost always cures the patient (Van Hagen 1956). Although this modality is generally in disfavor, it is an excellent tool when used correctly and should not be neglected because of its negative image.

SCHIZOPHRENIC EQUIVALENTS

Pain, usually of a bizarre nature, is one of the few equivalents that schizophrenic patients might have where the underlying condition would not be initially recognized. Any time the word *bizarre* is used about the symptoms of a patient, schizophrenia should immediately be included in the differential diagnosis.

> A 36-year-old Caucasian woman who had recently emigrated from the Netherlands with her husband and four children was referred to me by an orthopedic surgeon because she was taking too much Demerol. She "overcomplained" of her ter-

rible back pain, which not even the large amount of Demerol helped. She was taking 20 cc a day with 50 mg per cc subcutaneously, which is itself bizarre. That fact, when paired with her complaints, led me to the diagnosis of schizophrenic equivalent.

Her history revealed that the family moved to Southern California because her husband, a scientific technician, could make a better living there than in Holland. However, during their first year in California, one child drowned in a neighboring swimming pool, while another was killed by a truck. My understanding of these traumatic events was that her environment had become too dangerous. I also felt that it was useless to try the phenothiazines. I therefore advised them to return to their native country. When they deplaned in Amsterdam her pain was gone. Because she did so well, they returned to Southern California six months later and the pain returned upon landing in Los Angeles. She returned to the orthopedic surgeon who removed a nucleus pulposus from her lumbar spine, which gave her no relief. The patient was placed again on ever higher doses of Demerol, and was soon referred to me a second time.

In a bizarre manner, she crawled into my office on hands and knees even though she was wearing a back brace. After talking with her, I immediately "ordered" her back to her native country, but the family was now without money. Several of the charitable agencies finally enabled them to make the move. Again, on landing in Amsterdam, she was without pain, and remained so for at least the next five years as revealed in her Christmas cards to me.

ATYPICAL FACIAL PAINS

Another rare condition, which belongs to the schizophrenic equivalent group, is that of atypical pain in the face, which is often misdiagnosed as tic douloureux or some other recognizable syndrome and treated accordingly and unsuccessfully. The pain is bizarre. The phenothiazines or other antischizophrenic medications will often control it. A therapeutic test can be applied, for the pain will usually return if the medication is discontinued, and then go away on reinstituting the medication.

SOMATOFORM PAIN DISORDERS (NEUROTIC EQUIVALENTS)

This condition has been known for years as one of the neurotic conversion symptoms, a class of conditions that commonly confuse physicians. It is usually diagnosed by nonpsychiatric physicians by exclusion; however, it is easily recognized by most mental health professionals because of other signs and symptoms. One of the most important symptoms is contained in the French phrase *la belle indifference.* It is seen in patients who present signs of a severe debilitating condition, including pain as in the following case, but seem to be grossly underreacting to that condition. They sometimes even act as if nothing is wrong. This defense is usually accompanied by "gains" for the patient in relation to life and family. It also exemplifies the symbolism of the actual symptoms.

> A 29-year-old single Caucasian woman was referred by her primary physician because of severe pain in her right shoulder and arm. She met me with a smile as she explained that her arm hurt too much to shake hands. Her history revealed that she lived alone with her elderly, and moderately senile mother. She also explained bitterly that her three older brothers and sisters could not understand why she was upset with the living arrangements. I knew before asking that the mother would brighten on the arrival of visitors, for that is the nature of moderate senility. I also found that the brothers and sister did not want to pay money for the kind of care that was really indicated.
>
> Dynamically, this young woman was very angry, but so "sweetly" unaware of this subconscious anger that she wanted to strike not only her mother but also her brothers and sister. This was characterologically impossible for her to even contemplate, so she converted this anger into a symptom that both punished her for the hidden feeling and made it impossible for her to make any motion that could be interpreted as a gesture toward hurting anyone

while keeping the forbidden anger below awareness. Since it was impossible for her to continue to do the housework, the condition also forced the issue of finding an acceptable place for her mother. Over a period of two months, her work with me in psychotherapy made it possible for her to find a new independence that she had never realized until then, and the pain evaporated.

IATROGENICITY

An inadvertent remark or gesture can cause some patients to develop a pain syndrome unlike any of the above conditions. The responsible person is usually a doctor, who does not do this consciously. A remark, often out of context, is interpreted by the patient as a pessimistic one about his/her condition. The patient will unconsciously overreact until s/he is sick, and the puzzled doctor will usually not understand. For example, in the operating room when the patient is under anesthesia, the only explanation for a stormy recovery from what had appeared to be an uncomplicated operation is that the patient was hearing the procedings. Cheek (1959, Cheek and LeCron 1968) proved conclusively that this not only happens, but that hypnosis can take the patient back to the operating room, so to speak, to find what the remark actually was. It is unfortunate that many physicians are still unaware that an anesthetized patient hears these remarks, even though in deep anesthesia.

> When I was stationed in Germany as a medical officer ten months after VE day of World War II, a 17-year-old girl was brought to my dispensary. She had been found "unconscious" beside the Autobahn, writhing in pain from a supposed heart attack. She claimed to be an American who had visited her grandparents before the war and was not able to return to America. Further questioning revealed the history of a traumatic experience at the age of 13, which involved a Nazi soldier scratching a swastika on her left chest with a bayonet and telling her that from that time onward, she would have a bad heart. There was a faint scar on her chest, and her heart was normal. I saw her only this one time and referred her to the German medical clinic.

Although the psyche and the soma are so interwoven that we have difficulty differentiating them, the conditions discussed in this chapter show how the psyche can unconsciously affect the body and vice versa. As with most conditions, the interweaving of the mind and body must be untangled, even though we know that they are a whole, in order to properly treat our patients.

PAIN AS A SOMATIC MEMORY

Since this is not a recognized condition, I introduce it here for completeness, for some books are now asserting that it is not just the brain that remembers. Some authors believe that the molecules in our body have memories (Freedman 1992, Gabbard 1992, Rossi and Cheek 1988, Tsuchiya and Williams 1992). Studies pointing only as far as the tissue area are as reductionist as necessary for me to understand this category of pain patients. I believe that a former trauma, occurring at an early age and repressed because it was too overwhelming to live with in conscious memory, can be "remembered" later in the tissues of the injured but healed area without conscious memory of the trauma. A future involvement of the area in question can cause the return of the pain, which usually persists steadily or sometimes episodically when there is nothing physiologically wrong.

> A 44-year-old Caucasian unmarried woman was referred to me by a neurosurgeon because of the uncertainty of the diagnosis. She had received injuries to her cervical and lumbar spinal areas from several auto accidents, but did not have enough pathology to warrant surgery. She had recently lost both of her parents through terminal illnesses; her three brothers were expecting her to do all the work about the estate, but were interfering. As she saw it, her life was useless, and she knew that she was also depressed. After a few years of intermittent psychotherapy, including hypnotherapy that helped her with her dental work but not her spinal discomforts, I realized that she resisted hypnotherapy because of unconscious conflicts about her life

situation. During the time when we were working out many of these conflicts, she fell and received a stellate fracture of her right patella. Although the knee healed well, she continued to experience severe pain in her knee. Regression under hypnosis revealed that she was hit by an automobile at the age of 5 with a resultant fracture of her right femur. Her hospital treatment included not only the traction of that leg but also the restriction of her parents' visits. This was not unusual in the late 1930s, but she experienced it as desertion. She had to wear a body cast for almost a year, and suffered much humiliation from her peers. Our interpretation was that the fracture of her patella, which occurred during a highly emotional era of her life, brought back to the tissues of her knee and leg the pain she experienced at the age of 5.

A 29-year-old Caucasian married woman sought treatment because of depression, her life being in disarray, and because of pain in her right shoulder, back, and neck. This was found to be in conjunction with left eye lachrymation. Her pain occurred only when she was thinking about her mother and stepfather and their very abusive relationship with her. With regressive hypnotherapy, a particularly brutal beating by her stepfather at the age of 8 came to light. He hurled her against a cabinet from which she received painful injuries to the area presently in discussion. When this episode, which was consciously remembered but not connected consciously with her present symptomatology, was associated, both the pain and the unilateral opposite-sided crying ceased. Other than when thinking of her parents, she had always cried in the normal bilateral manner. (This case is fully presented in LePage and Schafer 1994.)

11

PATIENTS WITH MULTIPLE PAINS

There are many patients who have simultaneous pains in different parts of their bodies. These patients must be carefully questioned about the origins of each individual pain. Many times the patient will give a history and background description of each pain that shows they have different origins and meanings. I estimate that 5 to 10 percent of my pain patients have had multiple pains of this nature. A physician must be suspicious and use careful interrogation to delineate them. The differences between these pains in the same patient involves both organicity and symbolism. These pains are not usually treated individually because of the law of parsimony. This law states that patients do not usually have more than one condition at a time; therefore, all the symptoms presented by the patient must be from a single source. The following patients with multiple pains prove this law has exceptions.

> A 34-year-old Caucasian, married bookkeeper and mother of two children by a former marriage was referred for pain in the right ovarian area that had lasted for three years. The cause was yet to be determined. Her pain seemed to start one or two days prior to her menstrual periods which were irregular enough that it was thought not to be anticipatory pain. This pain would last several days past the end of her period and was described as dull, heavy, and aching. She also had dyspareunia, pain during intercourse, as a second pain. Careful questioning left me with the conclusion that the marriage was good and therefore not involved in the causes of either pain. She stated that she was orgasmic. The first pain was controlled with minor narcotics and usually without absence from work. She had an exploratory laparotomy and tubal ligation two years earlier. She had a pelvic laparoscopy about four months after the first operation with reported normal findings. Birth control pills seemed to lessen the pain when they were used to correct some of the irregularity of her periods as well as interperiod spotting. She reported a "nervous breakdown" eight years previously which included a suicide attempt by overdosing. Her brother had been killed in a single car accident as a possible suicide near the time of her first operation. She had

three attacks of pericarditis at the ages of 17, 19, and 21. Cardiac investigation at the Scripps Clinic was reported to be negative as to pathology. Another pertinent diagnosis made by that institution, and therefore a third type of pain, was spastic colitis associated with periods of abdominal cramping and tenderness not associated with her ovarian pain, although it sometimes was concurrent.

The most important observation that I made of this attractive woman during her first visit was her Pollyanna attitude. Although she had experienced more than her share of troubles, including the divorce of her parents when she was young and her own unsuccessful first marriage as well as the above-stated difficulties, her life was subjectively remarkably good.

After obtaining the historical details of her life, which later included the description of a few headaches as a fourth type of pain, probably mild vascular ones, hypnosis was utilized and she was taught self-hypnosis including the use of the solar plexus maneuver (see Chapter 4). After six to eight visits, her colitis with its gripping pains was well under control. She spontaneously used self-hypnosis in the dental chair. She was not coached by me in this accomplishment, having used it from my previous treatment. However, her ovarian pain remained unchanged, and during her next visit it was in progress. This disappeared while she was in hypnosis in my office, but was not successfully controlled subsequently with self-hypnosis. Meanwhile, she maintained her Pollyanna attitude, which finally wavered at the end of the next meeting when she acknowledged that her husband did drink a little too much, eat too much, and have a somewhat edgy temper. Subsequently, he requested a therapist and soon began to see one of my colleagues on my referral, and I then began conjoined therapy with the husband and wife. As we solved their marital problems, she relinquished her Pollyanna attitude and made no more complaints of her ovarian pains or dyspareunia.

A 35-year-old married Caucasian man, a post office janitor with a master's degree in fine arts, presented symptoms of two types of headaches. One was a rather general headache of the vascular type that involved the entire head, the other was a severe typical tension headache that was bilateral and involved his neck and ran up over his head.

He was a quiet man from a quiet family. He and his four siblings were married to "screamers." He was severely wounded in the abdomen in Vietnam. He was addicted to Darvon compound because of his headaches. He admittedly took ten to twelve capsules for the rush feeling that he would then have. When the Veterans Administration changed its rules and he could no longer procure this medication by mail, he overcame this addiction with moderate withdrawal symptoms, but with no change in his pains. He has been on no medications since that withdrawal episode.

His headaches would appear separately or together. Hypnosis did not help very much although he appeared to be a good subject. Rather conventional analytically oriented psychotherapy revealed that his vascular headaches were connected with his identity crisis that was triggered by a car accident that occurred on his way to his parents' home after a delayed honeymoon trip to Europe. Further, this accident triggered a delayed posttraumatic stress disorder associated with his Vietnam wound experiences. He had worked for several years as a film and television scriptwriter, but became self-defeating with his vascular headaches, to the extent that he finally had to stop writing and take a job as a post office janitor.

His tension headaches were explored dynamically and it was found that his wife was the "pain in the neck." (This type of interpretation of body language was examined in Chapter 5.) His wife became involved in conjoined therapy and his neck-aches became almost nonexistent. His vascular headaches improved, but they did not stop entirely until his identity crisis and posttraumatic stress disorders were worked out psychodynamically.

A 33-year-old married, Latin American man, who had specialized in outdoor utility company work until placed in a responsible office position because of a pain disability that precluded physical work, was referred for left kidney area pain that did not respond to treatment. In describing this pain, he revealed that it had an anniversary origin, for he had an operation in October in each of four successive years. The first one was an irrigation of his left kidney for what he described as sand in it. The next year the kidney was removed. The third year a hernia in the area of the kidney operation was repaired, and the fourth year the hernia was again repaired with the use of nylon mesh. After this, as near as can be told on physical examination, he had an intact left side.

He had always been action oriented and actively engaged in athletics. His wife had an excellent office position and they had three children whom the patient enjoyed coaching in activities such as Little League baseball. The company that employed him was very understanding, arranging his switch from outdoor work to office work, and tolerating much absenteeism because of his pain.

He described four aspects of his painful kidney area. The first was that he had a rather wide, large, and tender scar that when slightly irritated gave a deep ache leading to an even deeper aching pain, exhaustion, vomiting, and several days in bed. His second pain was of a sharp nature in the scar area, which he would get if he twisted his trunk. This pain would last several hours, but would go away. The third sensation was that of an uncomfortable phantom kidney feeling. The fourth was of a burning type of pain, which I considered to be causalgic. As stated previously, I consider any burning pain to be evidence of autonomic nervous system dysfunction.

The third and fourth pains responded very quickly to hypnotherapy and autohypnosis control. The second pain, the sharp one upon twisting, was controlled also very well with a posthypnotic suggestion that his unconscious would help him protect that area automatically by preventing sharp turns and by splinting the involved muscles. The first pain, that of the severe deep ache on rubbing the scar, took a great deal of time before he had some relief. It was finally revealed that he felt he was unloved by his wife. In turn, she felt neglected by him. As a consequence, he felt very guilty and angry and retired into his pain and his bed feeling deeply miserable. When these aspects of his life were worked out in conjoint therapy, he improved rapidly and when last seen had been working approximately nine months without time off for sickness. The previous year before referral to me, he had spent almost half of his time off work.

When questioned closely, many pain patients have separately identifiable pains. Each pain may have a different meaning and require different treatment. It is important to "dissect out" these pains when using hypnotherapy or any other approach. Additionally, hypnosis helps in the diagnosis of these patients and in assessing which pains can be helped and which cannot without further dynamic investigation. This leads to better treatment of the patient by taking into consideration not only those different pains themselves, but also as they reflect the patient as a whole person in his/her milieu. These three cases are presented to illustrate many of these differences with special emphasis on the personal dynamics involved in some of the pains, the psychosomatic aspects of others, and the overall human situation that must be considered before treatment can be successful through the patient's history, physical examinations, and current relationships.

12

PEDIATRIC HYPNOTHERAPY OF PAIN

Children experience pain differently from adults. It is not that their neurological system is different, although it may be incompletely developed in the newborn; rather, it is that children do not interpret the world or experience pain as adults do. I treated two teenage boys who were burned in a fire. They were in a constant panic state, which was not helped with large doses of narcotics. This panic made it impossible for me to gain rapport with either of them and therefore defeated my use of hypnosis.

The older the child, the more likely the pain will be recognized, but even older children will distort what they say they are feeling in order to avoid getting an injection or something else that they fear will also hurt.

Once the condition of pain is recognized, the problem of treatment may be approached, even though most children also fear that the treatment will be inflicted on them and cause more and different pain.

It is more difficult to recognize when an infant is in pain. In the past it was thought that babies did not feel pain because of the incompleteness of their nervous systems. It was also thought that even if they felt pain, they would not remember it. This is a serious issue and should be examined from both positions, for we do not want an infant to experience pain if something can be done about it. There is much evidence now that children do remember even if it is kept from consciousness, for the experience may be so overwhelming that it is repressed. It can later come out of repression, sometimes as a somatic memory or as a neurosis. However, some patients actually do remember.

> A 45-year-old obese Caucasian unemployed business manager who was on welfare was undergoing psychotherapy with me for a *DSM*-diagnosed condition called borderline syndrome. Rather incidentally during one of his therapy visits, he described a consciously remembered incident that took place at his age of 9 months. He was taken to his family doctor for an office circumcision. His description of the sudden burning and excruciating pain was consistent with my knowledge of the use of a Gomco clamp procedure.

In my experience, many borderline-type patients have memories that extend back before the age of 5 or

6, when most of us have our memories begin. Conscious memory before that is sketchy and usually assumed to be screen memories. Psychoanalytic theory postulates that the ending of the Oedipus stage of emotional development is the point at which memory usually starts. Because of distorted oedipal circumstances in the infant who will become a borderline personality, the pre–6 years memories are often consciously preserved.

Roark (1991) reported that young sufferers are not receiving medicine to ease their pains, and that researchers are finding that unrelieved torment poses serious health consequences. A premature infant needed an extensive surgical procedure on his chest, heart, and lung, and it was done without any analgesia or anesthetic. This infant died a few weeks later although the operation was "successful." Roark reported that this was standard procedure in most of this country six years previously. She reported on the research that proved the experiencing of pain in newborns as well as in older children, and she detailed the advances in pain control from infancy to the age of puberty.

Most pain conditions are understandable through the neurological concepts of acute pain. The pain conditions for which hypnotherapy is indicated are caused by trauma, including operations. Terminal illnesses with painful treatments must also be considered. However, chronic, career pain is rare in childhood.

Adolescents are semi-adults, but their life is complicated by the turmoil characteristic of this age. In primitive cultures, they are considered adults after the puberty rites. In our culture, they cannot be adults, yet they see themselves as adults. Their conflicts modify their hypnotizability, but if motivated, they are excellent subjects.

Nor should we neglect helping the child in good health who must receive regularly scheduled injections that are experienced as pain inflicted by the doctor or nurse. This can result in a child becoming "allergic" to a visit to the doctor's office. A good hypnosis maneuver for children who must receive shots is to give them a "magic spot." This is accomplished by having a child go into hypnosis and telling him/her that before getting a shot s/he is to ask where it is to be given. That child is then told while in a trance that the next time he is to get a shot, either index finger is to be placed on the spot that is to have an injection. This will produce a fifty-cent size magic spot of numbness so that nothing is felt. It is amazing to see a formerly screaming and reluctant child go into the doctor's office and proudly ask that the shot be given "here." Furthermore, s/he does not have to be restrained. It is unfortunate that only a few hospital wards dedicated to treating very sick children do not have someone on their staff to help them with this kind of pain control.

Pain accompanies many childhood illnesses and can be dealt with individually with whatever hypnotherapeutic actions are indicated, for example by the use of direct suggestions for relaxation and comfort. There should be a good-enough rapport with the responsible adults, including the treatment personnel, to allow the child to experience his symptoms enough so that s/he can describe them to both the parents and the physician.

Children are hypnotizable from the ages of 3 or 4. It is probable that they are *conditioned* to obey their elders to such a degree that hypnosis is easily induced. Infants may be hypnotizable. Doesn't a mother's lullaby put her baby into a "trance?" Cuddling and soothing actions help a great deal. However, hypnosis in the early age group probably cannot be used for anesthetic purposes, which require verbal communication.

For the older child and in a situation where the hypnotherapist feels that rapport is good, a classic adult-type induction is seldom used. One of the reasons a less formal induction can be used is that children love to be in imaginative situations. This characteristic can be used for the induction as well as for the added suggestions that are considered necessary.

My usual routine is to inquire about the child's favorite television cartoon program. This requires that the therapist be knowledgeable about the programs (a good excuse to occasionally watch some of the Saturday children's shows). While the child is sitting in a comfortable chair, or lying as comfortably as possible in bed, I ask him/her to close the eyes. I then state, "With your eyes shut, you can see that TV. Now I am turning it on and your favorite program is there. And it is your program so you can make it happen just like you wish. And while you are watching and enjoying it, I'm going to tell you some things and another part of your mind will hear me, but you go right on enjoying your program." I then make whatever suggestions are indicated. During this session, it is not unusual for the child to open his/her eyes and glance around before immediately closing them again. Nor is it unusual for fidgeting to take place. The hypnosis actions are not like those of an adult. Specific directions for the control of pain, bleeding, healing, sleeping, and so on can be given before the child is told to end the TV program and come out of hypnosis feeling rested and comfortable, "when I snap my fingers." I will also give instructions about the proper use of self-hypnosis before dehypnotization. Some of the more common conditions for hypnotherapy in children are as follows:

ACUTE TRAUMA

Milton H. Erickson (1959) treated a 7-year-old boy with a bad cut on his knee. Erickson's approach was first to get his attention diverted by concentrating on how red the blood is. He used the sibling rivalry situation by wondering if this little boy would get more stitches than his older brother when that brother was previously injured. By the time they got to the emergency room, the boy seemed interested only in if he would be getting one hundred stitches, and did not seem to feel any pain in the wound or from the stitches.

> This case history may be apocryphal, but it does illustrate the situation. An 8-year-old boy was brought to the emergency room because of an extensive laceration of his neck and arm. He was in a panic state and thrashing and screaming on the stretcher. As the personnel were getting ready to restrain him into immobility, an enterprising intern asked for a moment with the patient. To get the boy's attention, he dabbed his finger in some of the blood and smeared it on the patient's nose. The surprise brought the panic to a stop and hypnosis suggestions helped him be an ideal patient.

The following procedures are applicable to many trauma situations and are very valuable if the child has a full stomach; chemical anesthesia can therefore be avoided. In the cases of burns and plastic surgery where many short procedures are indicated, hypnosis again can obviate the use of anesthesic agents in patients of all ages but especially children because of their excellent hypnotizability. Additionally, it can help control bleeding as well as help healing and keeping patients comfortable.

PHANTOM LIMB SENSATIONS

Krane and Heller (1995) state that most children and adolescents who experience amputations have phantom sensations, usually with pain. This is refractory to all treatments. However, hypnotherapy is, in my experience, the approach of choice (see Chapter 7).

HEMOPHILIA

Some attacks of hemophilia start with a spontaneous bleed into a joint, especially of the knee. Over time, this can result in severe injury to the structures of the knee, eventually interfering with walking. In Chapter 4, I describe in detail the transfer of the migraine spasm of the muscles in the blood vessel walls into the hand as a fist is made. This maneuver is reversed in the case of any bleeding in hemophilia so that the spasm of the clenched fist muscle is transferred into the bleeding vessels, especially of the knee so that the transferred spasm stops the bleeding. This is also explained in Chapter 4 as the reverse migraine maneuver. If the patient is too young to do this in autohypnosis, a parent can be taught to do it with the child. This procedure is pseudoscientific, but it works because the unconscious mind understands it. The skepticism of the family doctor, if told of this success, can negate any hypnotherapeutic maneuver done for a child, so the hypnotherapist must prepare the child and the family to try to prevent this from happening. If the child is scoffed at, the symptoms may return.

ASTHMA

This condition, in children, is more easily treated with hypnosis than it is in adults. The child's vivid imagina tion is the hypnotherapist's ally. I again ask children to see the television with their favorite program while I talk to another part of their mind. I explain the *end bulbs* in their lungs, which hold air in because something is squeezing the exit shut. I then tell them that they can loosen what is clamping it off and feel comfortable with the air going in and out freely, and that they do not need to have their asthma any more. This usually is effective in a very few visits, especially if the parents are supportive.

DENTISTRY

Hypnosis with the proper posthypnotic directions usually removes fears of dentistry as well as discomfort for the child. This is especially helpful in children with emotional problems. Additionally, there can be control of dryness of the mouth, the gag reflex, and bleeding, which can be life-saving in the case of hemophilia. (For further information see Kroger's [1977] section on pedodontics.)

MIGRAINE

This condition is fairly rare in children, and never before the age of 8 to 10. The dynamics are probably the same as with adult migraine patients (see Chapter 5). The treatment would probably include psychotherapy with much focus on family therapy. The migraine maneuver should prove effective, but not until the dynamics are understood.

CANCER PAIN

Hypnosis is very valuable in controlling the pain of cancer treatment. Not only can the pain of most treatments be eased, but many of the other effects of the disease and its treatment can be reversed. The "magic spot" is valuable for the many injections that the patients receive, and it is especially valuable for bone marrow aspirations, a procedure usually performed on the crest of the ilium, usually in leukemia patients. The nausea and vomiting seen with the x-ray and chemical treatments are usually relieved to a great extent with hypnosis and posthypnotic suggestions. The usual poor appetite can also be helped. The actual pain of this disease can be not only upsetting but also intolerable, and it can often be controlled. Hypnotherapy is therefore indicated for a large range of symptoms connected with cancer. Helping the child accept a realistic attitude toward the disease promotes a better self-hypnotic control of the symptoms as well as physical and emotional comfort, even in the terminally ill. Olness (1981) studied 25 cases where hypnotherapy was very productive in handling symptoms of cancer and cancer treatment symptoms. Gardner and Olness (1981) and Hilgard and LeBaron (1984) have given detailed advice on the use of hypnosis for children with cancer.

13

HYPNOTHERAPY AND PAIN IN THE ELDERLY

To consider the place of hypnotherapy in the practice of geriatrics, we must apply certain generalizations. From experience, we know that a 9-year-old child is more easily hypnotized than a 70-year-old adult. We also know that certain induction procedures work better in different age groups. But generally, hypnosis is applicable to all age groups.

When dealing with the older patient, we must recognize that when what there is in us that unconsciously selects the time and circumstances of our death may never be fully understood. Clearly the genes as well as other factors are also involved. Emotional conflict is an essential part of this equation especially when a person is "too young to die." As we get older, we can see our final illness as finishing our lives rather than solving an otherwise unsolvable conflict. The latter, I believe, is what we see in younger patients (Schafer 1984a). Statistics show that the two most common causes of death in the elderly are a neoplasm and the sludging up of an artery.

Many symptoms remain as some kind of complicated conditioned response after they are no longer dynamically needed. This is especially true of the aged who may have had their symptoms for many years. I would much rather try to help a migraine patient who has had the symptoms for 20 years than for 3 years. The latter will probably have a dynamic need of the symptoms, but the former no longer unconsciously needs the symptoms and is ready to accept relief. I find this is true with most of the classic psychosomatic illnesses, pain syndromes, and many of the phobias.

Kroger (1977) stated:

> Posthypnotic suggestions, in responsive persons, can effectively raise the aged patient's confidence and help direct thoughts from himself to external events; this can minimize depressive reactions and hypochondriasis. The suggestions also can help establish closer interpersonal relationships; many are quarrelsome, hostile over their infirmities and envious of younger and more agile persons.
>
> Definitive suggestions potentiated by hypnosis can be directed to: (1) taking an interest in the plans of younger persons (in this way the tragedy associated with the loss of friends or a mate is reduced); (2) developing avocational interests concerned with creativity, the acquisition of special motor skills, cultural activities; (3) exercise as walking, as much as possible; (4) watching the diet and the weight; (5) correcting elimination; (6) overcoming insomnia; and (7) physical in-

volvements, as cardiac congestion, arthritis and neuromuscular involvements. [p. 339]

GENERAL APPROACHES

Here are some givens in treating all adults, including the elderly.

1. Regressive techniques and hypnoanalysis can be utilized to explore symptoms.
2. The transference and countertransference situations are somewhat different in the elderly, especially if there is a large age difference between the therapist and the patient. But the hypnotherapeutic relationship fosters and intensifies both the transference and the countertransference. In this context, a 30-year-old male therapist can be a mother or father figure to a 70-year-old (Ferenczi 1955). It is also probable that the elderly are more interested in cognitive discussions of their problems; however, some elderly may be too set in their ways.
3. The susceptibility scales (Stanford Scales for Hypnotic Susceptibility) indicate that the aged are more difficult to hypnotize (Weitzenhoffer and Hilgard 1959). I do not believe that these scales have a place in clinical work; however, more preparation and explanation are needed to develop rapport and the motivation required for hypnotherapy in this age group.

4. An older patient probably has a stronger or healthier ego, unless the psychiatric history shows otherwise. But people do learn to live with their neuroses and are therefore not as motivated. The older patient does not seem to "give up control" as comfortably as the younger one, although experts in hypnosis know that this belief that control is given up is a gross misunderstanding and/or simplification believed by many people.

5. Autohypnosis, if indicated may be more difficult to teach to the elderly. Therefore, the use of a tape recorder is indicated more often than with younger patients. The patient can reinforce the hypnosis with the tape made in the therapist's office. On the positive side they have many more "safe places" or "havens" they can use for visualization and self-relaxation for their self-hypnosis.

6. It is not understood whether early senile changes (including Alzheimer's and dementia for other reasons) preclude the use of hypnosis. With stroke victims, the side affected may be important. If hypnosis is mostly a right brain function, then an insult to the right brain may make hypnosis more difficult.

DISEASE ENTITIES

Disease entities are handled essentially the same way as with younger patients when utilizing hypnosis. This section discusses diseases prevalent in the elderly.

Angina Pectoris and Intermittent Claudication

An angina pectoris attack is a signal to the person to stop everything. By realizing this, a hypnotherapist would never try to stop the pain as such. The same is true of the older person who can walk only a short distance before his legs hurt so much that he has to stop. However, hypnotherapy can be very valuable in such cases. After the patient is in hypnosis, the therapist can offer a guided image of lying in the sun on a warm day and "feeling" the (involved) blood vessels dilating. Of course, nothing will open a clogged artery or remove the cholesterol deposits, but this maneuver can help the vessels dilate and not only prevent spasms but also stay open wider because of the "feeling" of warmth in the chest and/or the legs. Additional posthypnotic suggestions that these individuals live within their abilities and that they use the visualization several times a day have helped several of my patients.

Also there are some therapeutic beliefs that the visualization of a large molecule cholesterol "animal" eating the small molecule cholesterol that is sticking to the walls of the arteries may at least somewhat reverse the atherosclerosis.

Visualization with a person whose circulation in the lower legs is so bad that gangrene is beginning, whether or not claudication is present, again involves feeling the warmth of the sun dilate the arteries of the extremities. This is indicated only in the earliest cases of gangrene, which is life threatening.

Peripheral Neuritis

This is a condition that can occur in several illnesses that are common in the elderly, such as diabetic neuropathy, severe vitamin deficiency, pernicious anemia, and sarcoidosis.

A symptom complex that is more apt to occur in the aged is hyperesthesia – a sensitivity to light touch – as well as lightning pains that are instantaneous, repetitive knife-like pains, especially of the upper body. The following case illustrates the hypnotherapeutic approach.

> A 64-year-old retiree with diabetic neuropathy was sent to me by his son, a physician friend of mine. He entered my office and immediately took off a fleece-lined jacket, the only clothing that he wore above his waist. He stated that if a feather would touch his chest, it would throw him into a spasm of pain. Additionally, "lightning pains" would attack his chest at irregular, but frequent intervals. Clearly the anticipation of these pains was as bad as the actual pain, which would last only a brief moment. It soon became apparent that he also could not renounce these pains because he needed them to tell his doctors how he was doing. I learned that he had been a cowboy in his youth. He explained that when he was riding a horse and something startled it, the horse would end up on the left side of the trail while he would be in the midst of a cactus patch on the right side. As a result of this, he was always alert. I induced hypnosis by having him

ride his horse to a campfire with two of his fellow cowboys at dusk, help prepare supper, get into his bedroll, and go to sleep. Although appearing to be in hypnosis, he continually would raise his head and open his eyes and then close them again. I proceeded as if he were fully hypnotized (which I think he was) and told him that the superficial pain would stop and he could elicit its equivalent only by deep pressure. I added that he could forget his lightning pains until one happened and then it would be over so quickly he would barely notice it before it was gone. This time distortion of the lightning pains plus the changing of his superficial pain into deep pain satisfied his needs. He was able to wear his normal clothing as well as go fishing and thereby enjoy his last three years of life.

Postherpetic Neuralgia

This pain syndrome often follows herpes zoster, or "shingles." It seems that the older one is when attacked by shingles, the more severe the pain is and the longer it lasts. Shingles is caused by the chickenpox virus that had been dormant for years. This condition and its treatment are discussed in Chapter 9.

Osteoarthritis

The wear and tear of aging is involved in the gnarled hands of older laborers, but I see the severe cases of this condition as primarily involving stress, reflected somatically in constant and mild tension of the muscles. This was discussed in Chapter 8.

There are other kinds of arthritis that must also be considered. Traumatic arthritis is like osteoarthritis but it is restricted to the joint near an old injury. One of the most common is the "football knee." This is also fairly common in the spine after disk surgery, and should be anticipated. Unless a spur impinges on a nerve, not unusual in the cervical area, the pain is the only problem. This can then be treated with "transfer of anesthesia." One of my patients was an ex-Olympic shot-putter with traumatic arthritis in his right hip. Since this condition was not made better or worse by any activity, at his request I taught him to use self-hypnosis and pain control so that he could enjoy mountain climbing.

Rheumatoid arthritis is also treatable by dynamic psychotherapy reinforced by hypnotherapy (Schafer 1994b).

Trigeminal Neuralgia

This is tic douloureux, a facial tic with lance-like pain that occurs mostly in older people. It was discussed in Chapter 9. There is very little in the hypnosis literature about this condition. Shafer (1962) describes two cases treated by autohypnosis, with self-induction of anesthesia of the appropriate index finger and using that finger as a "syringe to inject Novocain" into the affected part. He accomplished complete and permanent cure of his two patients.

Neoplastic Diseases

Most cancers are not painful until the terminal stages. The exceptions to this rule involve cancer of the pancreas or cancer of the bone. Although I feel that there is a place for the psychotherapeutic and hypnotherapeutic treatment of cancer (Schafer 1994a, Simonton et al. 1978), most hypnosis treatment is done to control pain as well as some of the symptoms associated with chemotherapy and other methods of treatment. The October 1982 issue of the *American Journal of Clinical Hypnosis* is devoted to the hypnotherapeutic treatment of cancer patients.

Sacerdote (1966) reviewed the literature on cancer pain control with hypnosis. He contributed a great deal to the use of hypnosis in the control of terminal cancer pain as did Erickson (1966).

Trauma

Since older people are more prone to fall and break bones, hypnosis for pain control is often very valuable. It contributes to the control of pain, but the patients must not see the doctors as trying to rob them of their needs, for example of analgesics and narcotics. Hypnotic suggestions will also help their peace of mind, as well as their healing and rehabilitation, if they are motivated. Posthypnotic suggestions to be more careful in their physical activities can be helpful.

Miscellaneous

For the patient in a terminal illness, the empathic closeness encouraged by the hypnotherapeutic relationship may lead to a smoothing of their final days. Many times the dying patient, especially with pain, just needs someone to understand and to talk to. The hypnotherapist, who may have been called upon to help control the pain, will establish quick rapport and can provide solace and understanding. I find that these patients want to talk about their coming death, but very few are willing to talk to them about it. This includes many of the physicians involved in their treatment. However difficult a task this is, I consider it a necessary part of our profession.

A transplant patient may have difficulty accepting the new organ. Preparing such a patient for surgery with hypnotherapy can include encouragement for the acceptance of the organ, which is now an integral part of his/her body. Direct suggestions for the body to accept the new organ may also be effective. As long as the patient experiences the new organ as foreign, rejection of that organ is likely. I have observed that the older the patient, the less likely that patient is to accept the new organ.

Dental patients can be helped by hypnotherapy to accept new false teeth.

The elderly who are on blood thinners can sustain bruises that may become severe hematomas. Hypnosis with the proper posthypnotic suggestions can alert them when they are bleeding and help control that bleeding.

14

TREATMENT

Treating the pain patients (acute, acute recurrent, and chronic) is one of the most important roles of a physician. Other health professionals are more limited in treating pain. It is important that the physician not automatically give medications just because the patient is demanding them. I have found that it is very difficult to treat patients with pain syndromes when they are misusing narcotics, tranquilizers, antidepressants, and other medications. This seems to be particularly true if some area of the body is already criss-crossed with surgical scars, or is the complications of arachnoiditis caused by previous intraspinal testing procedures or traumas. The most important rule, therefore, is that some patients will never be well, but we may be able to help them at least partially. And we must never feel omnipotent enough to think we can get 100 percent "cures" of any condition, let alone something related to pain.

Many physicians have become fixated in their treatment of patients by using almost exclusively the *acute treatment* approach. This approach is not applicable to most of the chronic diseases, which are the current problems in the field of medicine, because the chronic-career type of pain does not respond to analgesics and narcotics as acute pain syndromes do. When medications are used with the acute recurrent pain patients, it is symptomatic treatment only, which helps but is not curative. Health professionals who cannot prescribe medications are able to consider chronic diseases without the pharmacological mind-set. They have made many of the advances in the understanding of chronic pain (Hilgard 1975, Sternbach 1974).

HYPNOTHERAPY

Acute pain is often quickly controlled by hypnosis and self-hypnosis, especially if the pain can be anticipated. No treatment of pain, acute or chronic, should be instituted until the pain has been investigated as completely as possible—this includes the use of hypnosis. The patient who does not succeed clinically when hypnosis is used is usually "telling" the physician that s/he needs the pain dynamically and/or that something underlies the condition that needs to be diagnosed properly. Paradoxically, the patient who has dynamic needs involving his/her symptoms is often amenable to hypnotherapy as an investigative tool. One of the most effective uses of hypnotherapy is in those acute pains that are anticipated, such as obstetrics, dentistry, post-operative pain, trauma, and particularly burns (Ewin 1986, Schafer 1975).

PHARMACOLOGY

If a medication is going to be used, a sufficient dose must be prescribed. One of the modern medical sins is to underprescribe. The jaundiced eyes of the different state medical examiners may account for some of this over-caution, especially with the constant threat of malpractice suits. However, Joranson (1995) writes that the intractable-pain treatment laws and regulations, both federal and state, are now developing guidelines for the use of opioids for intractable pain. Nevertheless, in situations such as terminal cancer, and/or the treatment of the suffering elderly, the fear of addiction should not be an impediment to adequate treatment. If necessary, for the safety of the treating physician, the use of the narcotics can be registered with proper state agencies. Also, the family should be appraised of the situation. This is not to advocate inundating these patients with substances that keep them in a terminal, half-anesthetized state unless this is warranted, which it can be if the patient and/or the family requests it. Conversely, there are many patients who prefer a clear mind even if they must endure some pain. Hypnotherapy is then indicated as a first line of defense, not the last. Opioid use in chronic noncancer pain will often cement the symptoms of the career-pain patient.

Other modalities for handling the pain must at least be tried, for the sake of the patient and the involved families. Many career-pain patients will not respond to any drug but will often insist on trying any and all of them, often at the same time.

The steroids and the nonsteroidal anti-inflammatory drugs including the antiprostaglandins have added a new dimension to the treatment of some pain syndromes for they attack pain at a new site.

The antidepressants, specifically the serotonergic and noradrenergic mixed types, seem to work best and have effects on rest and analgesia not associated with their antidepressant effect. A patient can be both depressed and have chronic pain, at which point sufficient medication must be used. The non-antidepressant activities of these medications labeled as antidepressants are also often effective with one-fourth to one-half the ordinary dosage usually needed in depression. They are therefore valuable in sleep disturbances and sometimes act as calming agents.

SURGERY

I have seen many failures in surgical procedures in which nerves and tissues are interrupted as a means of controlling pain when the acute (telegraph) model of pain was applied to chronic, career-pain cases. Even a prefrontal lobotomy, probably the ultimate surgical procedure for pain, does not remove that kind of pain. The pain, after this type of psychosurgery, does not seem to bother the patient any more; however, it is still present. As a final attempt to control a terminally ill patient's pain, this procedure might be considered, but most physicians would see it as radical unless nothing else gave the needed relief. The stereotaxic interruption of spinal cord tracts must also be approached with great care and used as a last resort. Often these maneuvers yield negative results, which only proves that many pain patients do not use a built-in telegraph nervous system with their pain syndrome.

ANESTHESIA

The treatment offered by anesthesiologists is ultra-scientific and proves successful in carefully selected cases. The treatment is usually done in progressive steps of trial injections that confirm the diagnosis and give temporary improvement before a final tissue-destructive procedure is done.

LOCAL INJECTIONS

Injections include nerve blocks, nerve destruction, trigger-point injections, and other "attacks" on local areas. Novocain-like local anesthetics, alcohol, steroids, and other products may be used therapeutically to relieve or destroy tissues in conditions that are causing pain.

COUNTERIRRITANTS

Transcutaneous electrical nerve stimulation (TENS) is produced by specially manufactured machines that a patient can be taught to use. It has been an excellent addition to our armamentarium in the fight against pain. The use of this modality was a direct outgrowth of the gate control theory of pain (Melzack and Wall 1965). Originally, some of these devices were implanted into the spinal canal; in many cases they were of great benefit when the patient was the one who regulated the amount and intensity of the pulses and vibrations. Today, most patients can be treated by the external applications of the electrodes to the skin surfaces via a TENS unit. If there is not too much skin irritation from the electrode jelly, this can be of great help. The results seem to occur by irritating or stimulating the large fibers in certain nerve trunks and thereby closing the "gate" on the pain impulses. However, all effort should be made to understand why the pain is present.

ACUPUNCTURE

Some pain experts see this modality as almost a magical treatment. However, Kroger (1973) considers this treatment as "hypnosis" wherein the needle stick acts as a method of induction. Others think that the needle is also a counterirritant, especially when electrical stimulation of the needle is added. It may also be a "safe pain," which diverts attention from the site of the pain being treated. The usual descriptions of the "force fields" and the "meridians" are pseudoscientific in my opinion. Many therapists agree that a cultural background involving an Oriental belief system contributes greatly to its success. In China, surgical patients are carefully selected for acupuncture. It is an excellent tool in only approximately 10 percent of their patients (Kroger 1973).

BIOFEEDBACK

Most modern biofeedback is based on muscle relaxation. Benson's (1975) contributions show that skeletal muscle relaxation lowers anxiety; therefore, any pain syndrome based on either muscle spasm or anxiety, or their combination, will be helped by the proper application of biofeedback. Disease involving the autonomic nervous system can also be improved by biofeedback. I feel that hypnosis is more versatile and is therefore a better approach. It does take more training to become a skilled hypnotherapist than a biofeedback technician. Teaching the patient self-hypnosis and thereby personal control also seems to me to be a better approach for most patients. Ideally, the patient will also be gaining valuable insight.

PSYCHOTHERAPY

Psychiatric treatment can do no harm except for the time involved. Unless the doctor is capable and willing to look at the whole patient in his entire milieu, he should at least have a consultation from a psychotherapist who may be able to uncover secondary gains that the patient is unconsciously utilizing. Unless these are recognized, the patient will probably not improve, regardless of any intervention of the above-listed procedures and medications. This statement applies to the chronic, career-pain patient and depends on a correct diagnosis. Since most of these patients have been suffering for years, a few months dedicated to an attempt at psychotherapeutic intervention cannot be considered too much of a risk. For this approach to be successful, not only the patient, but his family, job, commitments, and finances must be considered. If the patient can be helped to "de-stress" his/her life, the handling of the pain syndrome will improve or be relieved completely. If, additionally, the psychotherapist is an expert in the proper application of hypnotherapy for diagnostic as well as treatment purposes, a much better and quicker result will be forthcoming. Biofeedback and meditation may also be of great help, depending on the patient and the skill of the therapist. It is unfortunate that many chronic, career-pain patients have used up most of their money before getting to a psychotherapist.

HOSPITAL TREATMENT

A hospital ward specializing in the treatment of patients with chronic pain syndromes must be considered. From my observations, although these institutions claim to be multidisciplined, the usual approach is organic and behavioral. This is often very successful. However, the institutions will usually reject patients with recognized active primary or secondary psychological gains from their pain conditions. But to the pain-ward's credit, the approach with a "pain-medicine cocktail" that uses progressively smaller amounts of narcotics during hospitalization does not allow narcotics to interfere with the treatment routine for the patient. Within five to seven weeks, by using every modality the program has at its disposal, many patients are able to leave either with complete relief or at least the ability to mentally *compartmentalize* the pain so that a better life is possible.

ELECTROCONVULSIVE THERAPY (ECT)

Van Hagen (1956) detailed the use of ECT for intractable pain. An intensive, regressive treatment series succeeds in many cases, and is considered very safe by most experts using this modality. Careful follow-up is needed after discharge from the hospital, for the pain usually returns in a few weeks and is then controlled by two or three outpatient ECTs. Nine months to a year later, there is often another return of the pain, and again a few outpatient ECTs will suffice. This is usually the last of the pain syndrome. This approach seems to be rediscovered every fifteen to twenty years. In spite of the view of ECT as a primitive and outmoded procedure, it is a very valuable tool in psychiatric treatment. The bad "magic" of electricity and the patient's amnesia account for ECT's rejection by the public.

When ECT is used in treating intractable pain syndromes, its mode of action can only be speculative. Its advantages include the elimination of narcotics (which can be easily withdrawn during these treatments) and reversal of any depression or possibly schizophrenia, which may not have been recognized. There is also the possible interruption of a reverberating circuit that is maintaining the pain. Another theory is that the period of amnesia interrupts the memory of the pain so that the patient returns to his world without the pain. Those people who regard ECT as a primitive treatment might argue that the frightening experience only conditions the patient from having or complaining about the pains. However, an intravenous barbiturate anesthetic and a muscle relaxant are administered so that the patient does not subjectively experience any of the administration of the electricity. The negative symptoms produced by the ECT are reversed in a relatively short time, making this preferable to a tissue-destructive procedure.

OUTDATED REMEDIES

Some of the old remedies from yesteryear were all that were available at that time. Pain also was not as well understood as it is today. The use of poultices, cupping and wrapping with red flannel, may have had some effect both as placebos and physiologically. The use of heat and cold is now restricted either to immediate use in acute injuries or to the home remedy of the heating pad or liniments. These modalities may help in some of the minor ailments, but when they are not sufficient, a visit to the physician is indicated.

THE FUTURE

Regarding possible future discoveries several questions come to mind:

1. Will a narcotic-like substance be discovered that helps control pain without producing addiction? This has to be answered in the negative if a substance is found to act like the endorphins. But we can hope that something will be found, not only as a narcotic replacement, but also one that may help even chronic, career-pain patients. However, dynamically, what would that patient do as a way of defending him/her self when robbed of the pain?
2. Will health professionals, physicians in particular, be able to comprehend the mind/body whole? It is hoped that this will gradually come about. If the professional will learn the proper use of hypnosis as an added tool, I believe it will occur sooner. This would also lead to a better and more

cooperative spirit between the different groups of professionals in the health sciences.

3. Will a new diagnostic and/or treatment tool be found that will make the treatment of the pain patient quicker and easier? We can only hope so.

15

SELF-HELP

Health professionals must instruct patients to never try to self-treat a pain they do not fully understand! Treating it blindly could be a most dangerous action. As an example, a psychotherapist friend, who is very adept in his use of self-hypnosis, was troubled by an acute toothache but felt that he did not have time to do anything about it, and used his self-hypnosis with great success in controling the pain. Actually, he then forgot about the problem. Six months later, his visit to his dentist revealed that he now had to have extensive and costly work done on his teeth, which would not have been necessary at the time the pain started if he had sought dental help immediately. His pain sent him a real message.

SELF-MEDICATION

Most incidental pains can be handled by aspirin or Tylenol or the newer over-the-counter pain remedies, such as the antiprostaglandins, or NSAIDs like the ibuprofins. This will take care of common headaches, arthritic aches and pains, and other minor pain problems. However, any pain that lasts longer than expected must be investigated by a physician. Also, logic tells us that any pain not easily eliminated by the above medications should have professional attention. Heat and cold as well as massage and liniment may be of help. However, if the medications do not give relief in an unknown or not understood pain, the patient should see a physician immediately.

SELF-HYPNOSIS

Also referred to as autohypnosis, self-hypnosis can be of great help to many people with pain if that pain is properly diagnosed and therefore understood. However, it is difficult to learn self-hypnosis from a book. It is best to learn it from a licensed health professional skilled in the use of hypnosis. Once control of the pain is experienced in hypnosis, the patient can take over with autohypnosis. This self-hypnosis is then a way of lessening, or even relieving, pain. If the pain is an anticipated one such as for childbirth, dentistry, or approaching surgery, a hypnotherapist can help prepare for the event and the control of pain. Once a pain is understood, *no one should have to hurt.* With the help of a hypnotherapist, any motivated patient should be able to control pain. The previous chapters have discussed different aspects of pain and why hypnosis, acupuncture, biofeedback, and other altered state approaches might not work. If they do not, a health professional should be consulted.

In an acute situation (usually involving trauma) and one in which there is full, conscious understanding of the situation, including the pain, the first thing the patient must do is to *believe* that the pain is no longer really necessary. Once definitive treatment has been instituted, the injured person may be helped to relax by thinking of a pleasant experience. Most people think of a scene in their past such as sitting in a boat while fishing or resting in a mountain meadow. This is most effective if the person with the pain can be in as comfortable and safe a situation as possible; however, I have had patients placed in hypnosis in a seemingly impossible situation. For example, I have induced hypnosis on a noisy burn unit while the patient was in the middle of a painful dressing change, and I have also failed to do so under those conditions. Visualization is in a sense a conscious flashback to a picture of a happy time in life. If one is flashing back intensely, one is already in a partially altered or dissociated state. Most people can do this; however, some are more oriented in the sense of hearing or bodily feelings. If this is the case, it will test the ingenuity of the therapist to help the patient find the right setting. When visualizing that safe place or haven, it is important to include all of the senses. Also, relaxing the muscles is recommended. A visualization that I often use, and which anyone can use and modify to suit one's own need is as follows: After induction, I say, "Please know that you are now at your beach. You are lying on your blanket and have wiggled around so that the sand under your blanket conforms to your body, just right. You need not pay any attention to anyone else who might be there. Feel the healing rays of the sun on your body just relaxing you and making you feel good. See the beautiful water, the waves, the surf, and perhaps a boat or two. Notice the different blue of the sky, and perhaps a few fluffy clouds up there, and be so relaxed that you do not even feel like making any pictures in those clouds. Perhaps you can hear the soothing sound of the surf just lulling you into comfortable rest, as a noisy gull flies overhead. Smell the tang of the sea air, and even taste a little salt from the sea spray on your lips. Just be comfortable and relaxed so that you can heal as fast and as well as you can, and without difficulties. Trust your unconscious to help you and to take care of you." (If there is bleeding, I say, "You need not bleed any more than absolutely necessary.")

I instruct patients to do this several times a day and I often put it on an audiotape. This can be done with whatever scene in a safe place. It can do no harm and it may help immensely. The above visualization is only an example, for after all it must be a personal visualization.

The same can be done for chronic pain, but this

would be in a situation far different than an acute accident. The patient should be advised that it would probably be best to seek a health professional skilled in the use of hypnosis for pain problems that are amenable to hypnosis.

> A 50-year-old Caucasian college teacher was to take a trip to the Orient in two days when she scalded a silver dollar–sized area on the inside of her left wrist with what should have resulted in a third-degree burn. She did not want to go on her trip with bandages and other treatment paraphernalia, so she called her physician husband at work, who reminded her that she was familiar with Ewin's (1976) approach to third-degree burns, and advised her to use it. That evening, there was much redness of the area, the next day only a little, and at the time of departure, there was none. I observed all of this because the woman is my wife and an excellent hypnosis subject. She told me that her first visualization was a beach in Tahiti, but the water was too warm on her wrist, so she then placed herself on a surfboard I had built for the northern Great Lakes, with her hand in the cool water, where it felt comfortable and healing could take place.

Books

I have found very little help for people from most of the books on self-hypnosis. Those that might work usually involve such a compulsive and lengthy routine that the average person will not complete the book's instructions. Additionally, many people in hypnosis do not subjectively feel different, so they would not necessarily know that they had entered a trance state. If there is no immediate reason for learning the self-hypnosis advocated by the book in question, there is no real motivation, which is one of the cornerstones for the use of clinical hypnosis. *Motivation* is an abstract word, difficult to pin down to specifics. It can be as simple as being sick and tired of taking Tylenol. It can be used for insomnia, for there are very few people who do not enjoy having a good night's sleep. A person who is tired of tossing and turning night after night might be motivated to try hypnosis. Smokers may be similarly motivated to find a way to quit. Hypnotherapy works best with proper motivation.

I do not advocate books as a way of learning self-hypnosis. If it is important enough for a person to learn self-hypnosis, he/she should go to a licensed health professional who utilizes hypnosis and be instructed in its proper use. People who approach a hypnotherapist for theoretical purposes will not accomplish much unless they are specifically motivated. If there is a good reason for the hypnosis, success is much more likely.

16

SUMMARY

Acute, acute recurrent, and two kinds of chronic pain syndromes have been discussed in an effort to present an approach to the problem of pain and its treatment with hypnosis. Emphasis was placed on the need to distinguish these pains so as to conceptualize them and then to plan appropriate treatment for the specific pain situation. An effort was made to avoid the mistake of looking at chronic pain as either organic or functional. Both must be considered. Special pain syndromes where pain is the predominating symptom, not just the accompaniment of an otherwise well-known syndrome, were presented. These were described and special approaches were discussed. Hypnosis, as a tool, was emphasized in certain of the syndromes. It can be used diagnostically, prognostically, and/or therapeutically in almost all of the pain syndromes discussed. A plea was made repeatedly that the career-pain patient be treated as a whole person in his/her milieu, and that such a patient's pain cannot be treated with only the concepts of the neurological telegraphic model of acute pain. Information on this subject and names and locations of health professionals who use hypnotherapy can be obtained from the two hypnosis societies:

The American Society of Clinical Hypnosis, Arlene M. Stern, Executive Director, 2200 East Devon Ave. #291, Des Plaines, IL 60018-4534, phone (708) 297-3317.

The Society for Clinical and Experimental Hypnosis, Joyce Martello, CAE, Executive Director, 3905 Vicennes Road, Suite 304, Indianapolis, IN 46268, phone (317) 334-9470.

Both of these societies are accredited by the American Medical Association as providers of type I continuing education credits. Both have annual workshops and scientific programs as well as some local chapters. Their membership is made up only of licensed health professionals of at least a master's-degree level. There is also The International Society of Hypnosis.

I have presented the following ideas about pain:

1. Hypnosis success as well as resistance is useful for diagnostic as well as treatment purposes. Clinically, there is no such thing as someone who is

unhypnotizable. The patient will go into hypnosis under the direction of the hypnotherapist to whatever degree is necessary to accomplish what is desired. If not, it is not lack of hypnotizability—it is psychological resistance (see Appendix A).

2. Many times, symptoms should be regarded as merely conditioned responses. The original dynamics of the patient's unconscious are no longer active and patients are often ready to renounce their symptoms if they can be given proper control. Hypnosis is the best means of accomplishing this.

3. There is no such thing as generic pain. All pain has causes, but it may not be in the sense of the telegraph model of pain transmission and response still utilized by most physicians.

4. No one should have to have pain. However, both physical and psychological understanding of the patient is necessary to alleviate any specific pain.

5. The chief function of the autonomic nervous system is to control the caliber of the blood vessels. The ANS is very close to consciousness and can be manipulated by the patient through hypnosis. The reverse of this must be considered in the concept of negative self-hypnosis as a cause of many diseases.

Modern hypnosis is permissive and does not suggest that the hypnotherapist dominate the patient. The modern aim is for the patient to assume responsibility for his/her condition, with or without hypnosis and self-hypnosis. It is one of the safest tools that a therapist has.

APPENDIX A: THE FIVE STATES OF HYPNOSIS

My approach to hypnosis is that it cannot be defined and that we waste our time trying to do so. This appendix goes into detail about the different states of hypnosis as well as other variables that tend to validate my assertions. This theoretical material is not necessary for the understanding of pain and hypnotherapy.

INTRODUCTION

There have been innumerable attempts to define hypnosis since the concept of animal magnetism was rejected and this set of phenomena was termed

"Hypnosis" by Braid. Acceptable definitions have begun with "hypnosis is an altered state of consciousness" (Lynn and Rhue 1991).

These definitions then proceed to describe, rather than define, many aspects and phenomena we have associated with hypnosis. I strongly disagree with this approach. Hypnosis is neither a state nor is it altered consciousness. It is a composite of states; it is not necessarily altered consciousness. Many subjects/patients do not subjectively feel "altered" and objectively do not appear other than relaxed in the usual hypnosis situations. This appendix discusses the reasons for much of the confusion. Simply put, there are too many variables involved in hypnosis; as stated, it is not a single unified state, and traits and situations contribute to the number of variables. Hypnosis can no more be defined than can sleep or consciousness. This would imply that if we cannot define consciousness (or unconsciousness) it seems useless to use either in defining yet another term. I shall therefore list some of the variables involved in the trait aspects of hypnosis. I shall then do the same for the variables involved in the situation of hypnosis. Finally, I shall describe five states that appear to be intertwined in hypnosis. I will end with such a number of variables that it should appear obvious why a definition is beyond our reach.

My aim, therefore, is to try to stop the futile attempts to define hypnosis. Instead, I advise that we turn, by analogy, to something like quantum theory to derive further understanding of this thing that we call hypnosis.

TRAITS INVOLVED IN HYPNOTISM

All persons involved in hypnosis have traits. This applies to both the hypnotist and the subject/patient, but I shall focus on the subject/patient.

E. Hilgard (1965) states that hypnotizability is an inherited trait, that it is probably multigenetic and is comparable to the probable multigenicity of intelligence. This is undoubtedly true in the experimental laboratory. Laboratory studies indicate that this trait is relatively stable throughout the life of the individual. A personality trait that also seems associated with hypnosis was described by J. Hilgard (1970). She found that adults who as children had vivid imaginations were most hypnotizable. Wilson and Barber (1983) seem to validate this in their work with a group of women where the most hypnotizable were found to have the most vivid and most constant daydreams.

Liebeault and Bernheim (1957) felt strongly that the only important variable in hypnosis was the trait of suggestibility. Most experts in the field would probably agree that this trait is in some way intertwined with hypnotizablilty, especially in the clinical setting.

The Spiegels (1978) have associated a physical trait, the ability to roll the eyeballs upward, as an all-important factor in hypnosis and judging hypnotizability. That it is associated with hypnotizability in some way cannot be refuted.

The above traits may have developmental aspects also. One that may be associated with development, by definition, is the trait of age-related susceptibility. Children are seen as much more likely to enter hypnosis than any other age group. Conversely, age seems to rob many of some of this ability, at least in the experimental laboratory (Hilgard 1965). However, large aspects of this factor of age may be much more situational than trait involved.

SITUATIONS INFLUENCING HYPNOSIS

In the situations involving hypnosis, the hypnotist is at least as important as the subject/patient. This is maximized in the clinical area, and often minimized in the laboratory. The traits of the hypnotists as well as the overall situation will influence the hypnotizability of the subject/patient. The Freudians, especially Ferenczi (1955), conceptualized hypnosis as being an experience in fathering or mothering, which was not necessarily related to the sex of the hypnotherapist. This may also account for a probably related aspect: those people trained to react quickly to authority–especially soldiers, who see officers are "father figures"–are described as being better subjects (Hilgard 1965). Motivation of the subject as well as the hypnotist, whether it is seen as partially trait or situationally related, is seen by many hypnoclinicians as one of the most important hypnotizability factors in hypnotherapy. This becomes translated into some of the maneuvers of the hypnotherapist to influence a patient maximally as a prelude to clinical hypnosis and has prompted the concept of the clinical quotient (Schafer, this volume). Already the number of variables involved in hypnosis are seen to be too numerous to lead to an easy definition. So let me now introduce five more as intertwined "states" of hypnosis.

THE STATES OF HYPNOSIS

I propose to examine hypnosis as a variety of states combined into a composite, thereby giving different measurements compatible with the number, prominence, and combination of these states.

A beginning to this approach was made by Shor (1969), who viewed hypnosis as a single state with essentially three aspects. Semantically this may not differ much from my approach, but it does define these dimensions as aspects of a single altered state of consciousness.

This leads to another problem and another semantic difficulty. Are all altered mental states altered states of consciousness? This problem becomes most apparent in the alterations in autonomic nervous system function as seen in the field of biofeedback research, where it is obvious that some kind of altered mental functioning causes changes, but where subjectively and objectively there usually is no altered state of consciousness (see below).

One other difficulty concerns regression, which is recognized as one aspect of hypnosis. Differentiation must be made between semi-voluntary regression, age regression in hypnosis, and forced regression as observed in many cases of psychopathology. Some clarification came with the concept of regression in the service of the ego as developed by Hartmann (1958) and as applied to hypnosis by Brenman and Gill (1961).

The reader may be wondering if I am trying to group together all recognized altered states and conditions and call them hypnosis, including even transcendental meditation and acupuncture. The only answer to this is a very qualified yes. It is my impression that most of these so-called altered mental states, especially those effected without drugs, are found in that condition called hypnosis and are found in certain mixtures with the other states under discussion. This is not to say that acupuncture is hypnosis, but it does suggest that acupuncture can be at least partially comprehended by viewing it as an altered mental state or states, similar to some found in hypnosis. Hypnotic anesthesia must be very similar to the anesthesia in acupuncture, but without the use of needles in hypnosis or a formal induction process in acupuncture. There is some agreement by others, including Wall (1972) and Kroger (1973), the former an expert in the understanding of pain and the latter an expert in hypnosis. Agreeing with Kroger (1973), the endorphin studies at Stanford, associating those opiate-like substances with acupuncture, appear to me to be too simplistic in their implications. Subsequent studies have found that the endorphins do not play a part in hypnotizability (Barber and Mayer 1977, Finer and Terenius 1981,

Goldstein and Hilgard 1975). The reader may also wonder if I am labeling attributes as separate states. I am cognizant of this difficulty and the fine line of distinction. For example, hypnotic anesthesia is recognized as an attribute or phenomenon of hypnosis, but the regression found in hypnosis is, I believe, a combination of two states identified by their particular attributes, as explained later.

One final critical question must also be faced: Can these so-called separate states be identified and examined? I think they can as long as we realize that it is as artificial as identifying the *psyche* and the *soma,* for those terms represent a whole or a continuum that we artificially break up solely for the purposes of examination and further understanding. These attributes, as described by Shor, which I consider to be states, must now be described.

State of Deautomatization

This state, for which Shor credits White (1941), is an altered state of consciousness, in my estimation the only one we will see. Several descriptive adjectives can be utilized but the word *deautomatization* is the one used by White. This word implies that the hypnotized person, to a greater or lesser degree, puts aside those mental processes that supply him automatically with the sense of orientation. A person in so-called deep hypnosis can be disoriented as to time, place, and/or person. At the same time s/he has set aside at least some critical thinking (Aristotelian logic). The concept of depth is appropriate to this state only and not to the others. Depth in hypnosis is usually measured vertically by the amount of deautomatization. Also, most of the phenomena measured in hypnosis susceptibility scales derive from this state, which is also experienced in hypnogogic and hypnopompic situations and is subjectively experienced at the point of transcending the world in meditation. It is also described in religious ecstasy and certain mystic experiences. It has many facets in common with pathological conditions involving depersonalization and estrangement, especially in schizophrenia; but to equate that kind of a mental illness with conditions that occur in healthy individuals goes beyond the scope of this book, as does comparing some of those phenomena with ones produced chemically in drugged states. When we do a mental status examination, we in essence are looking for changes that occur in this state, but we are really looking for psychopathology, not a voluntarily entered state that we call hypnosis.

State of Role Playing

Shor credits Sarbin and Coe (1972) for their investigation of hypnosis as an unconscious role-playing phenomenon. Shor felt that this is measurable along a continuum from conscious role playing to a state where the role is so automatically played as to be out of consciousness. Actors sometimes assume the personality of the part they are playing, often past the time of their stage presentations. The fact that this process can be taken past the point of conscious role playing has led to much confusion in the literature by those who need to demean hypnosis as predominantly an artifact if not a fraudulent state. Phenomenologically, each subject utilizes his/her own understanding of hypnosis, taken from observations and the myths of culture, to perform a role that is felt to be required. The many facets that can be brought to this performance accounts for much of the variation observed by workers in the field of hypnosis and for much of the skepticism of observers who are often not knowledgeable in this field.

The final attribute proposed by Shor concerns the more primitive unconscious feelings the subject has for the hypnotist. I have divided this attribute into two states, one of action and the other of thought.

Transference State

Dynamically oriented therapists would call this state of unconscious or more primitive action *transference,* but it is usually not handled therapeutically as it would be in classic psychoanalytic treatment. In most hypnotherapeutic situations neither the therapist nor the patient is aware of transference as such, although the therapist should be. The exception to this is in hypnoanalysis. The hypnosis relationship is considered by most to be very intense and empathic. *Rapport* is another term that is used to describe this interpersonal state. Kline (1958) equates hypnosis with transference. On the other hand, Meares (1965) uses the word *atavistic* to describe this more as a state than as a process. It is seen in other conditions, such as mob action. Freud (1930) connoted mob action with hypnosis and described the primitive thinking evidenced by the mob that reacts under the direction of a leader. It is important, however, not to carry the comparison too far, because, as Freud said, the superego or conscience is neglected in mob action when people allow themselves to be directed to do things they otherwise would not. While in hypnosis, the subject does not negate any aspect of his mind, will not act contrary to his own conscience, and is in a position of trust and belief not found in the mob scene. These two words, trust and belief, are therefore basic attributes of this interpersonal state of transference.

The concept of basic trust need not be elaborated here other than to mention that if it were not present there would be interference with the intensity of hypnosis, whether on the conscious or unconscious level. The word *belief* is even more subjective although closer to consciousness, and involves the subject thinking it is safe to allow him/herself to be directed by the hypnotist. Both edges of this sword are involved, first that the hypnotist is to be trusted, and second, that the subject will act within character (whether the hypnotist is or is not worthy). Much of the understanding and misunderstanding about hypnosis is an outgrowth of trust and character. Although thought and action cannot be totally differentiated in this context, it is felt that transference relationships are better understood in the sense of unconscious action, that is, acting out behavior, than in ways of thinking, which seems to refer more to the next state involving regressed thinking.

Shor proceeded to mathematically combine these three dimensions of hypnosis—deautomatization, role playing, and transference. I consider these separate states in order to demonstrate the varied aspects of hypnosis observable in both the clinic and the laboratory.

Additional States

I feel there are at least two additional states that further influence and help explain the varied observations of this condition called hypnosis. These concern the special state of regressive thinking (the second part of Shor's third attribute), and the state of function of the autonomic nervous system. Both states are primarily under the control of unconscious forces and cannot be measured in the sense of depth.

State of Primitive Thinking

The state of regressive or primitive thinking is not as difficult to describe as it is to differentiate from other conditions involving regression, for this term has been applied principally in three different ways. First, sick regression is probably best known and refers to patients, usually sufferers of mental disease, who are forced, as part of their illness, to rely on previous or regressed methods of thinking in order to cope with the world because some of their more mature defenses have failed.

The second concerns a phenomenon of hypnosis

called age regression, which extends from hypermnesia, to seeing the previous event, to reexperiencing the previous ego state. This is one of the most utilizable characteristics of therapeutic hypnosis (Schafer 1981), and it must be differentiated from the other two phenomena of regression.

However, the concept of regression in the service of the ego as forwarded by Hartmann (1958) and discussed in application to hypnosis by Brenman and Gill (1961) is a partially voluntary and temporary condition and is based on the confidence of the ability for that individual to return to his normal mature state. It is also characterized as being positive, either in the sense used by Berne (1961) when one indulges his "child," or therapeutic when utilized in a treatment setting. It is always reversible and usually has an element of conscious choice.

Third, to further differentiate primitive or regressed thinking from sick regression and age regression and help its conceptualization as a state, we can comprehend it as a condition where thinking is of an ativistic or a more primitive kind. It is this more primitive thinking that also distinguishes the state of regression in the service of the ego from the transference state, although these two states intertwine in the sense of trust and belief. In the transference situation, patients act toward therapists as they had acted toward significant individuals in the past.

Therefore, this state reveals earlier methods of thinking, manifested by concrete interpretations of words and other evidence of what psychoanalysts call primary process thinking. The more the primary processes are utilized, the more intense the state. It is necessary for the hypnotherapist to understand depth psychology.

State Involving the Autonomic Nervous System

The autonomic nervous system is much more difficult to see as a state, for it requires either instrumental measurements of its functions or the removal of symptoms to infer that a change has taken place. In other words, the person who is "in" an altered autonomic state usually does not subjectively feel altered. Investigators in the area of biofeedback phenomena have utilized this state (which has also been manipulated at times in hypnosis) in their research. Unfortunately, the clinical hypnotists who utilize this state to alter autonomic nervous system dysfunction report their material anecdotally. It is probable that the changes can best be measured clinically in psychosomatic illnesses like migraine and asthma. Thus, until the researchers in biofeedback arrived on the scene with their sophisticated measuring instruments, the potentials for altering these autonomic changes were either not recognized except in the field of hypnosis or, even worse, were ridiculed. However, the problem seen here (in addition to advocating that the techniques of the experimental laboratory be applied in clinic settings with publishable proofs) concerns the dimensions of this state and those that appear to have evolved from treatments aiming at relaxation but not necessarily recognized as hypnosis.

Schultz (1932) and Luthie (1970) in Germany and Jacobson (1938) in this country have used autogenic training and progressive relaxation as their main therapeutic tool in the psychosomatic illnesses. Liebeault and Bernheim (Bernheim 1993), in the second half of the last century, and Meares (1971) have utilized hypnosis to attain this same kind of relaxation. Although relaxation is probably the most common denominator of the condition called hypnosis, and a pathway to effecting these normalizing changes in the autonomic nervous system, the translation of the skeletal muscle relaxation to relaxation of the smooth muscles of the bronchial tree, for example in asthma, was anything but clear until Benson (1975) documented his work on the relaxation response. Also, it is obvious from the findings in biofeedback that there is much more to the autonomic changes than just relaxation, which may be a pathway to normalization of autonomic pathology, but cannot explain changes away from the normal. When this is understood, a great step will have been taken in clarifying psychosomatic concepts, for somehow we must have initially mentally produced any pathological changes that can be therapeutically reversed by hypnosis, relaxation, and/or biofeedback. The concept of negative unconscious self-hypnosis adds to our understanding (Araoz 1985).

Therefore, we are talking about a state that is altered, that is involved in mentation via relaxation and other, as yet unknown, pathways, which probably involve the limbic lobe and/or the ascending reticular substance as well as higher centers. This state is not experienced as an altered state of consciousness for the patient does not feel "different." However, many measurements are changed in both the central nervous system and the peripheral organs. This is the reason I have utilized the term *altered mental state,* which seems most appropriate. Another difficulty concerns its measurements as a state other than through one of its attributes, physical relaxation. Via relaxation, we might conceptualize this as a state measurable by this attribute rather than by depth.

DISCUSSION

Because of the five states found in various admixtures in that condition known as hypnosis, it becomes apparent that a complicated set of variables exists. That is why so many varied findings have occurred in research aimed at examining hypnosis as a single state, a state of depth. It is felt that this approach also helps explain one aspect of the dilemma between experimental and clinical hypnosis. For years, clinicians have observed that there is not necessarily a direct correlation between depth of hypnosis and clinical results. Most measurements of depth deal with only the first state, that of deautomatization. We can now see that the fifth state, that involving the autonomic nervous system, can be altered for improvement in psychosomatic illnesses without a measurement of depth. The opposite may also be true, that a person "deep" in hypnosis will not necessarily be able to effect change in his autonomic nervous system.

There may be other conceptualizable states to add to these five, and when the other variables affecting hypnosis are combined with these five states, we realize what a complicated situation hypnosis really is and why a definition is impossible.

APPENDIX A REFERENCES

Araoz, D. L. (1985). *The New Hypnosis.* New York: Brunner/Mazel.

Barber, J., and Mayer, D. (1977). Evaluation of the efficacy and neural mechanism of a hypnotic analgesia procedure in experimental and clinical dental pain. *Pain* 4:41–48.

Benson, H. (1975). *The Relaxation Response.* New York: Morrow.

Berne, E. (1961). *Transactional Analysis.* New York: Grove.

Bernheim, H. M. (1957). *Suggestive Therapeutics.* Westport, CT: Associated Booksellers.

_____ (1993). *Hypnosis and Suggestion in Psychotherapy.* Northvale, NJ: Jason Aronson.

Brenman, M., and Gill, M. (1961). *Hypnosis and Related States.* New York: International Universities Press.

Charcot, J. (1962). In *Psychology in the Making: Histories of Selected Research Problems,* ed. L. Postman. New York: Knopf.

Ferenczi, S. (1955). *Selected Papers of Sandor Ferenczi,* ed. M. Balint. New York: Basic Books.

Finer, B., and Terenius, L. (1981). *Endorphin involvements during hypnotic analgesia in chronic pain patients.* Paper presented at the Third World Congress on Pain of the International Association for the Study of Pain, Edinburgh, Scotland, September 4–11. (In Barber, J., and Adrian, C., Eds. (1982). *Psychological Approaches to the Management of Pain.* New York: Brunner/Mazel.

Freud, S. (1930). *Civilization and Its Discontents.* London: Hogarth.

Goldstein, A., and Hilgard, E. (1975). Lack of influence of the morphine antagonist naloxone on hypnotic analgesia. *Proceedings of the National Academy of Sciences* 72:2041–2043.

Hartmann, H. (1958). *Ego Psychology and the Problem of Adaptation.* New York: International Universities Press.

Hilgard, E. H. (1965). *Hypnotic Susceptibility.* New York: Harcourt, Brace, & World.

Hilgard, J. R. (1970). *Personality and Hypnosis.* Chicago: University of Chicago Press.

Jacobson, E. (1938). *Progressive Relaxation.* Chicago: University of Chicago Press.

Kline, M. V. (1958). *Freud and Hypnosis.* New York: Julian Press.

Kroger, W. S. (1973). Acupunctural analgesia: its explanation by conditioning theory, autogenic training, and hypnosis. *American Journal of Psychiatry* 138(8).

Luthe, W., ed. (1970). *Autogenic Therapy, vol. 4: Research and Theory.* New York: Grune & Stratton.

Lynn, S., and Rhue, J. W., eds. (1991). *Theories of Hypnosis: Current Models and Perspectives.* New York: Guilford.

Meares, A. (1965). *A System of Medical Hypnosis.* Philadelphia: Saunders.

_____ (1971). *Demonstration.* Annual Meeting of Society of Clinical and Experimental Hypnosis. Chicago.

Sarbin, T. R., and Coe, W. C. (1972). *Hypnosis, a Social Psychological Analysis of Influence Communication.* New York: Holt, Rinehart, & Winston.

Schafer, D. W. (1981). The recognition and hypnotherapy of patients with unrecognized altered states. *American Journal of Clinical Hypnosis* 23(3).

Schultz, J. H. (1932). *Das autogene training.* Stuttgart: George Thieme Verlag.

Shor, R. E. (1969). Hypnosis and the concept of generalized reality orientation. Three dimensions of hypnotic depth. In

Altered States of Consciousness, ed. C. T. Tart, pp. 233–250; 251–261. New York: Wiley.

Spiegel, H., and Spiegel, D. (1978). *Trance and Treatment. Clinical Uses of Hypnosis.* New York: Basic Books.

Tart, C. T., ed. (1969). *Altered States of Consciousness.* New York: Wiley.

Wall, P. (1972). Acupuncture, an eye on the needle. *New Scientist,* July 20.

White, R. (1941). A preface to a theory of hypnotism. *Journal of Abnormal Social Psychology* 30:477–506.

Wilson, S. C., and Barber, T. X. (1983). The fantasy prone personality: implications for understanding imagery hypnosis and parapsychological phenomena. In *Imagery: Current Theory, Research and Application,* ed. A. A. Sheikh, pp. 340–387. New York: Wiley.

APPENDIX B: THE CLINICAL QUOTIENT CORRELATION BETWEEN HYPNOTIC SUSCEPTIBILITY DEPTH AND CLINICAL RESULTS

Robert C. Heidenrich
and Donald W. Schafer

A shorter version of this paper was presented to the 10th International Congress of Hypnosis and Psychosomatic Disease in Toronto, Canada on August 14, 1985. Clinical and experimental research cannot, in the opinion of most clinicians, be judged solely by the rigid standards of the experimentalists. This paper helps illustrate the difference between hypnotizability as measured in tests and as it appears in the clinical arena. The term *clinical quotient* is used to illustrate that the clinician considers and uses every aspect of the setting, the patient, the interpersonal relationship and anything else that will encourage the patient to benefit from that complex state that is called hypnosis. In this paper, pain is considered generically, without specific diagnostic categories, for this was a general experiment not focused primarily on one patient with one type of pain.

This paper presents a relatively unobtrusive experiment with 66 patients from the University of California, Irvine Medical Center Hypnotherapy and Pain Evaluation Center, who were chosen at random and tested with the Harvard Group Scale of Hypnotic Susceptibility Form A as they sought treatment and before the treatment started. During the treatment, and at the time of discharge, they were evaluated for depth according to the Orne-O'Connell Scale. A good correlation was manifested between the clinical results and the latter scale; however, each category (poor, fair, good, and excellent) as compared to the Harvard scale showed no significant correlation with the Orne-O'Connell Scale or the clinical treatment results. Details of the methodology and the concept of the clinical quotient that came out of this study are presented.

At the time of the study, Dr. Heidenrich was working as my student at the Hypnotherapy and Pain Evaluation Center. He was also working for his advanced degree. This study met in part the requirements for his Ph.D. in Psychology at the International College in Los Angeles and is taken from his dissertation. He is now the director of the Pain Evaluation and Reduction Center in Corona, California. We wish to thank our wives Viola Schafer and Dawn Heidenrich for their help; Susan Cooperman, Ph.D. for administering the Harvard scale to all subjects; Vikki LaBrecque, Ph.D. for her advice on the statistical aspects; Tim Ryan, Ph.D. for his thoughtful and perceptive comments on the dissertation; and Loren Sanders, for his editorial comments and help.

The tools of psychotherapy are numerous. The specific tool, hypnosis, is probably one of the least understood. One reason for this is that the laboratory setting for examining hypnotic phenomena is somewhat different from the clinical situation. The authors offer the concept of the clinical quotient to help explain some of these differences. We hope this will add to the understanding and additional use of the tool of hypnosis by therapists.

Experimentation or research in trying to explain the hypnosis phenomena did not occur until the mid-nineteenth century. Investigators, such as James Braid, Jean Charcot, Pierre Janet, Ambroise-Auguste Liebeault, and Hippolyte Bernheim, experimented within the clinical doctor–patient setting. Without benefit of modern statistical or research tools, some of these pioneers attempted to understand and explain hypnosis phenomena through neurological studies (Braid 1843, Charcot 1878) and psychological studies (Bernheim 1957, Braid 1843). Sarbin (1962) writes that Liebeault reported a 97% success level for hypnosis in 1,756 cases, and Bernheim an 80% success level in 10,000 cases. Perhaps they intuitively worked within the framework of what we are now calling the clinical quotient. It contains that set of variables usually limited by the experiments in the laboratory but utilized maximally by the clinician.

In the last decades, much attention has been given

to the measurement of hypnotizability, depth, and/or susceptibility. Because the measuring instruments were developed in the research laboratories, their relevance to the clinical setting has been debated by a number of investigators (Frankel et al. 1979, Hilgard 1979, Hilgard and LeBaron 1982, Perry et al. 1979, Sacerdote 1982). According to Perry and colleagues, "The result of this near universal belief among clinical investigators that hypnotic susceptibility counts for little in clinical settings has been until quite recently, a dearth of empirical findings addressed to this issue" (p. 141). However, credit must be given to Gruenewald (1982) for perhaps the most succinct and objective statement of the problems that fuel this debate. She emphasizes that clinicians use all variables available in hypnotherapy as contrasted with the laboratory attempt to control as many variables as possible.

To add to the difficulties, there has been major confusion caused by interchanging such terms as *hypnotic depth, susceptibility,* and *hypnotizability,* thus giving identical meaning to different terms (E. Hilgard 1969) and at other times attributing different meanings to a single term (Tart 1979).

Today we cite two scales/instruments used in the laboratory: The Stanford Hypnotic Susceptibility Scale, Form A (SHSS:A) (Weitzenhoffer and Hilgard 1959) and the Harvard Group Scale of Hypnotic Susceptibility, Form A (HGSHS:A) (Shor and Orne 1963). For this project, the most significant instrument for measuring actual hypnosis is the Orne-O'Connell Diagnostic Ratings of Hypnotizability (DRH) (Orne and

O'Connell 1967). The latter two tests are the ones used in this study. The DRH has been respectably correlated with the SHSS:A in the laboratory, and the SHSS:A and the HGSHS:A have been well correlated (Bentler and Hilgard 1963, Bentler and Roberts 1963, Evans and Schmeidler 1966, O'Connell et al. 1966, Shor 1969, Shor and Orne 1963). Although these correlations are not perfect, these scales represented the only tools available and were the ones best known to the authors.

In the clinical setting, the works of both Frankel and colleagues (1979) and Perry and colleagues (1979) dealt with correlations between the scores on the Stanford scales and independently assessed clinical outcome. In both of these studies, the testing was an integral part of the treatment.

The present study evolved from measuring hypnosis phenomena in the clinic in such a way as to explore similarities between the laboratory and the clinic. Tests for measurements used in the laboratory have been assumed by many clinicians to have the same measurement validity when applied to patients in the clinical setting. The inference is that a person with (laboratory) low hypnotizability would be seen as a poor (hypnosis) patient in the clinic and would probably not be considered for hypnosis intervention.

In 1982, the director of the clinic (D.W.S.) implemented the use of the HGSHS:A during the introductory group session for all new clinic patients. This was done for over a year and resulted in 131 HGSHS:A completed forms from January 1982 to March 1983. These tests were all performed by the same psychologist in groups of two patients or more. These tests were not scored at the time of testing. Also, during the course of supervision, the DRH was evaluated for each patient. Approximately six months later, the other author (R.H.) decided to utilize the material already gathered as a project for his dissertation. However, the files were not complete in about half of the cases. The only files not included in the project were ones that were incomplete–none was eliminated for reasons other than stated.

METHOD

Our hypothesis was that there would be a significant difference between the scores on the HGSHS:A and the DRH with pain and nonpain treatment groups and with each other when performed in a clinical setting. Additionally, our conjecture was that a laboratory scale might not be applicable in a clinical setting for either or both pain and nonpain patients. It was felt that motivation, which is different in the clinical setting, as well as other factors such as the transference, the archaic aspects (Meares 1961, Schafer 1980, Shor 1969), the setting modified hypnotizability. These are the variables included in the clinical quotient. The laboratory tries to control the variables so that it can best study only one aspect of hypnosis at a time. Except for the study by Hilgard (1979) in which approximately one-fourth of the healthy subjects showed increased susceptibility when positively motivated, there have been no studies of this variable of motivation. A paper on motivation and compliance by Orne (1966) states that results are not necessarily correlated with depth, for some patients in light trance can produce marked therapeutic changes. He also demonstrated the importance of the transference relationship.

With the supervisor and the student making the decision as to the placement of the patient on the DRH, bias is a possibility even with one author's (D.W.S.) years of experience with this scale. Special care was taken at the end of treatment so that bias would not enter as a pairing of results and depth. However, the ability to assess hypnotic responsivity in such a way that it is not seen by the subject as a test but rather as integral in the therapy session is very valuable and, it is hoped, offsets the biases somewhat. The patients were questioned about their experiences in hypnosis, but were not informed that this was any kind of a test. The DRH score reflected the deepest hypnosis reached by the patient during his/her treatment.

In assessing the statistics on those patients for whom six or more months had passed after termination of treatment as well as the recording of the DRH and the grade of success or failure of treatment, it was necessary to bring the HGSHS:A and the DRH scales into a more utilizable comparison so that each of the scores could be applied to the pain and the nonpain groups and to each other. The DRH was therefore extended to thirteen divisions by using the plus and minus signs. This gave a parallel to the twelve divisions of the HGSHS:A (Table B–1), which is not strictly accurate, but is felt to be quite close.

TABLE B–1.

Orne/O'Connell Diagnostic Rating Scale (OODRH)
and
Harvard Group Scale of Hypnotic Susceptibility Form C (HGSHS)

CONVERSION CHART

Orne/O'Connell Diagnostic Ratings of Hypnotizability OODRH Scoring Criteria	Converted to + and - Orne/O'Connell Scale (OODRH)	Converted Numerically Orne/O'Connell Scale (OODRH)	Harvard Group Scale Form C HGSHS	HGSHS Scoring Criteria
No Response	1	N/A	N/A	N/A
Response/Motor Suggestion	1+	1	1	Head Falling
Idemotor Response	2-	2	2	Eye Closure
	2	3	3	Hand Lowering
	2+	4	4	Arm Immobilization
Challenge Responsive	3-	5	5	Finger Lock
With Subjective Involvement	3	6	6	Arm Rigidity
Hallucinatory Responses	3+	7	7	Move Hands Together
	4-	8	8	Communication Inhibition
	4	9	9	Fly Hallucination
Amnesia	4+	10	10	Eye Catalepsy
True Posthypnotic	5-	11	11	Posthypnotic Suggestion
Response	5	12	12	Amnesia Not Complete
	5+	13	13	Amnesia Complete

See Orne and O'Connell 1967 and Hilgard 1965.

SUBJECTS

The 66 subjects in this study were from a university-staffed outpatient clinic, the Hypnotherapy and Pain Evaluation Center. All patients were voluntarily seeking pain relief or control of symptoms. All came from the general population with various income levels. The methods of payment included cash, insurance-reimbursement, and/or governmental support. All patients had to make some type of payment even if not from their pockets. No statistics were kept about this. Subjects were selected serially over a period of approximately one year. Their already collected records were divided into pain and nonpain categories to prepare them for statistical evaluation. Other variables known about these patients, but not presented in this study, were sex, age, and number of anticipatory sessions. Statistical analysis of these factors revealed no significant differences and were noncontributory.

This study was biased toward individuals who were consciously motivated to utilize hypnosis. They were also all English speaking (one deaf man was not included in the study). There was no direct observation of the patient–therapist diad. Because the therapists as well as the supervisor were unaware of the HGSHS:A scores, no bias was possible in that area. The final decision about the DRH rating occurred at the last supervision, at which time the rating for success of the treatment was also made. The measurement had been made by the student hypnotherapist in separate supervisory sessions with only one supervisor (D.W.S.). It was felt that there was a minimum of bias in this format, although the possibility is acknowledged. The hypnotherapists were all studying hypnosis at the center and were M.D.'s, Ph.D.'s, third and fourth year medical students, Ph.D. candidates, and marriage, family, and child counselors (either in a master's program or in possession of a license). All were instructed in the DRH. Finally, the teaching philosophy of the clinic asserted that any patient who came to the clinic for hypnosis treatment would go into hypnosis to whatever extent needed to accomplish what s/he came for. If the patient did not, this indicated psychological resistance, not lack of hypnotizability. This would count toward the bias that there were no 1's or 1+'s, and only one 5+ in the DRH scores. Also, the possibility of bias cannot be eliminated concerning therapist enthusiasm with deeply hypnotizable patients. Each therapist was instructed on how to utilize clinically all the variables that can influence the clinical setting. Furthermore, there may have been some cures due to other variables, not the hypnotherapy. For this paper, hypnosis is defined as a condition in a subject characterized by increasing responsiveness to the operator's suggestions. For clarity in the hypnosis situation see Kroger (1977).

PROCEDURE

The statistical data had been gathered from January 1982 through March 1983. The categories of hypnotherapists have already been described. All had nearly the same amount of training and study hours in hypnosis procedures. Levitt and Overley (1965) have shown that experience of the hypnotist is likely to be irrelevant to subject performance in a standardized research situation. The hypnotherapists were to do their hypnotherapy, make appropriate progress notes, and review each patient's case with the supervisor at least once a week. All aspects of the case were considered during supervision, including the DRH scores. The final DRH score was therefore a composite of the opinion of the hypnotherapist and the supervisor by the time of the patient's discharge. During supervision, the diagnosis and therapeutic approach to the patient was discussed. Although hypnosis was not used in each session, it was seen as the primary tool in this type of short-term therapy employing the supervisor's psychodynamic understanding of patients and their problems. Most students worked in the clinic one day a week for six months; a case load consisted of five patients. No one student saw more than five patients involved in this project.

Each patient was assigned at random to a treating hypnotherapist after the initial interview, during which the HGSHS:A was given. This test was performed during the first visit by the same individual whose duties were to administer the test and then present an introduction to, and answer questions about, hypnosis. The first visit was charged the same as all visits at an hourly rate. The patients were not told the results of their testing, but only that it was a test of hypnosis. All tests were done in a group setting and utilized a tape recording that had been made from the booklet that accompanied the test packet. All of the scoring was done at least one year later by an author (R.H.) without prior knowledge of the results. The patients were seen by the treating hypnotherapist from a minimum of two to a maximum of seventeen treatment sessions, with a mean average of seven. No more than eight sessions could be utilized without the prior permission of the supervisor. The 50-minute sessions were usually held once a week. The patients were told that there would be eight sessions or less and that no follow-up was possible. The results were determined by the therapist and supervisor as poor (no change in symptomatology), fair (some definite changes, but not enough to satisfy either the patient or the therapist), good (definite change with satisfied patient and therapist, but not complete), excellent (no residual symptoms). Not only did the treating hypnotherapist keep the usual records required for a modern clinic, but the supervisor kept notes on a file card, which also contained the DRH estimation.

All subjects for which complete data were collected (66 out of 131) were treated by hypnotherapy for their presenting complaint. They were divided into two main categories of primary complaints: pain and nonpain. In this study, the definition of pain is *an unpleasant hurting sensation experienced as physical in nature and occurring in varying degrees of severity*. Causes may be attributed to either physical or emotional trauma, some examples of which are headache, spastic colitis, and neck or back pain. Nonpain is defined as a physical or psychological disorder or symptoms lacking a physical hurting sensation, which is ego dystonic and varies in degrees of severity. Examples of nonpain complaints are altered consciousness-like states, smoking, phobias, habit disorders, impotence, weight control, and poor self-image.

Of the original 131 patients in this study who were given the HGSHS:A at the initial interview, as well as an explanation of hypnosis and the rules and limitations of the clinic, thirty-nine did not return for their next scheduled appointment and therefore received no treatment, as such. Clinically, it was felt that many of these thirty-nine patients had appeared at the urging of significant others and/or for "magical" cures, and therefore did not return. Of the remaining ninety-two patients, data from twenty were not used because of incompleteness of their records. We were unable to make contact with the previous treating hypnotherapists to achieve record completion. Finally, data were utilized from seventy-one patients (forty-eight female and twenty-three male). Thirty-eight were in the pain category and thirty-three were in the nonpain category. Since all patients came to a *hypnosis* clinic, none refused hypnosis. Since the use of the more powerful parametric tests as opposed to nonparametric tests (Elifson et al. 1982) requires an equal number of subjects in each group, five patients from the pain group were randomly dropped from the original seventy-one using a computerized random number generator. The final series of patient data used numbered sixty-six, with thirty-three in each of the two groups. The statistics were gathered without a project in mind at the time of testing, and they had lain fallow for six or more months before this project was conceived.

RESULTS

There was marked significant improvement (good and excellent) shown in 61 percent. A total of 85 percent showed significant improvement (excellent, good, and fair). Only 14 percent showed no improvement (poor).

Distribution or frequency of the HGSHS:A and DRH scores tend to show both the DRH and the HGSHS:A curves to be a bell shaped leptocurtive curve. The DRH mean score is 6.9 and median score is 7. The curves of the HGSHS:A mean score is 6.9 and median score is 7, thus giving the DRH a slightly more negative curve. The curves of the HGSHS:A and the DRH curves in each treatment category seem otherwise equivalent (Figure B–1, Table B–2).

Kihlstrom and colleagues (1980) gathered over a five-year period six samples ranging from 42 to 110 subjects. Their overall mean was 6.9 on the HGSHS:A, which was the same mean for this project.

A two-by-two factorial design analysis of variance (ANOVA) was used to test the differences between the HGSHS:A and the DRH scales, the pain and nonpain patient groups, and the interaction between the scales and the groups. To summarize, the two-by-two ANOVA and the required F-ratios showed that at a .01

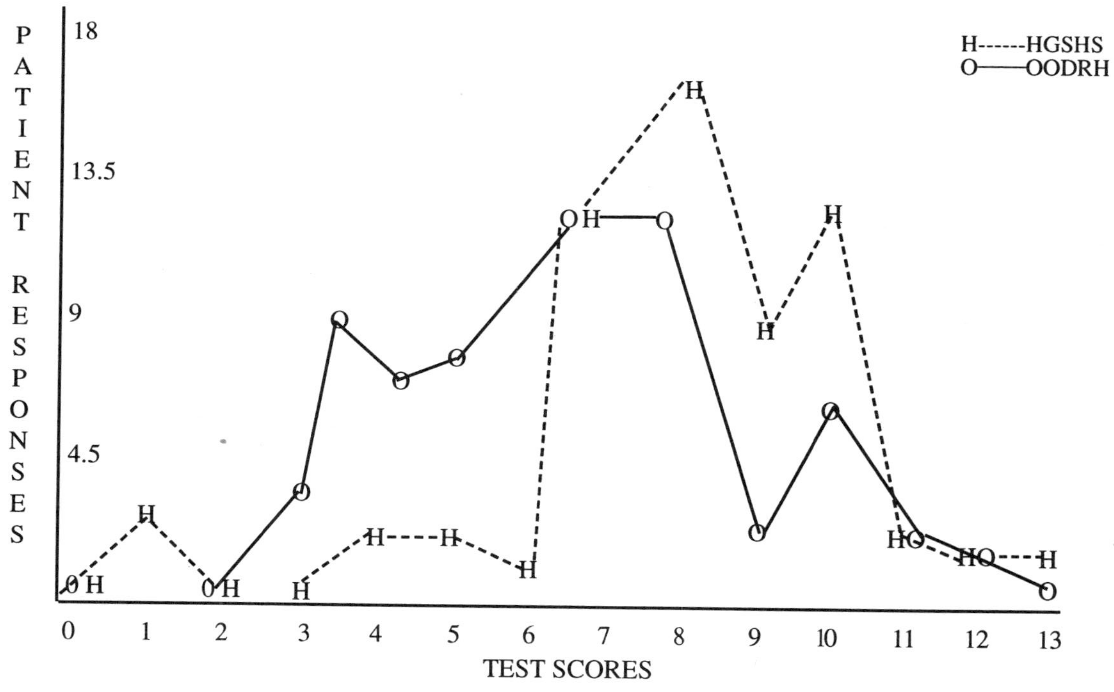

Figure B-1. OODRH and HGSHS Response Curves

TABLE B–2.

Distribution of HGSHS and OODRH Scales
with Treatment Results

	1=Poor		2=Fair		3=Good		4=Excellent		Totals	
Score	HGSHS	OODRH	HGSHS	OODRH	HGSHS	OODRH	HGSHS	OODRH	HGSHS	OODRH
1	0	3	3	0	0	0	0	0	0	3
2	0	0	0	0	0	0	0	0	0	0
3	0	0	1	0	2	0	1	0	4	0
4	1	2	1	1	2	0	5	0	9	3
5	0	1	2	1	2	0	3	1	7	3
6	2	1	2	1	2	0	2	0	8	2
7	2	2	5	5	4	2	1	3	12	12
8	3	1	4	6	2	6	3	4	12	17
9	0	0	0	0	1	4	2	5	3	9
10	1	0	1	2	2	4	3	6	7	12
11	1	0	0	0	0	1	2	2	3	3
12	0	0	0	0	0	0	1	1	1	1
13	N/A	0	N/A	0	N/A	0	N/A	1	N/A	1
Tota'	10	10	16	16	17	17	23	23	66	66
Mean	7.50	4.40	6.90	7.00	6.40	8.60	7.08	9.10	6.90	7.90

level of significance there is no reliable difference between the two main effects (Figure B–2): group (A) pain and nonpain patients, and the scales of group B1 and B2 of the HGSHS:A and DRH. However, there is a reliable interaction (A × B) (Figure B–3). With a significant interaction present in the ANOVA, a further analysis was made by comparing the two levels of one factor at each separate level of the other factor (Huck et al. 1974). This was found to be redundant (Table B–3).

To further this analysis, comparisons of the HGSHS:A and the DRH were made as to outcome of treatment in both the pain and nonpain groups. The instrument used for this analysis was the biserial correlation. The treatment categories were dichotomized as positive treatment results noted or no positive treatment result noted. The first dichotomy (positive treatment results) included the fair, good, and excellent categories; the second (the poor treatment results) included those patients showing no improvement following treatment.

Results of the biserial correlation (Table B–4) indicate that at a .05 or less level of significance, there is a correlation between the DRH scores and the treatment results in both pain and nonpain groups. However, no significant correlation was shown for the HGSHS:A and treatment results in either group.

In this study, the results of the two-way analysis of variance showed no significant differences between the pain and nonpain patient groups with regard to overall test scores. The DRH and the HGSHS:A scales tended to show no significant difference by interpolating the ANOVA of their respective scores. With an $F = 4.85$,

FIGURE B–2.

PLOT OF INTERACTION BETWEEN OODRH AND HGSHS SCALES

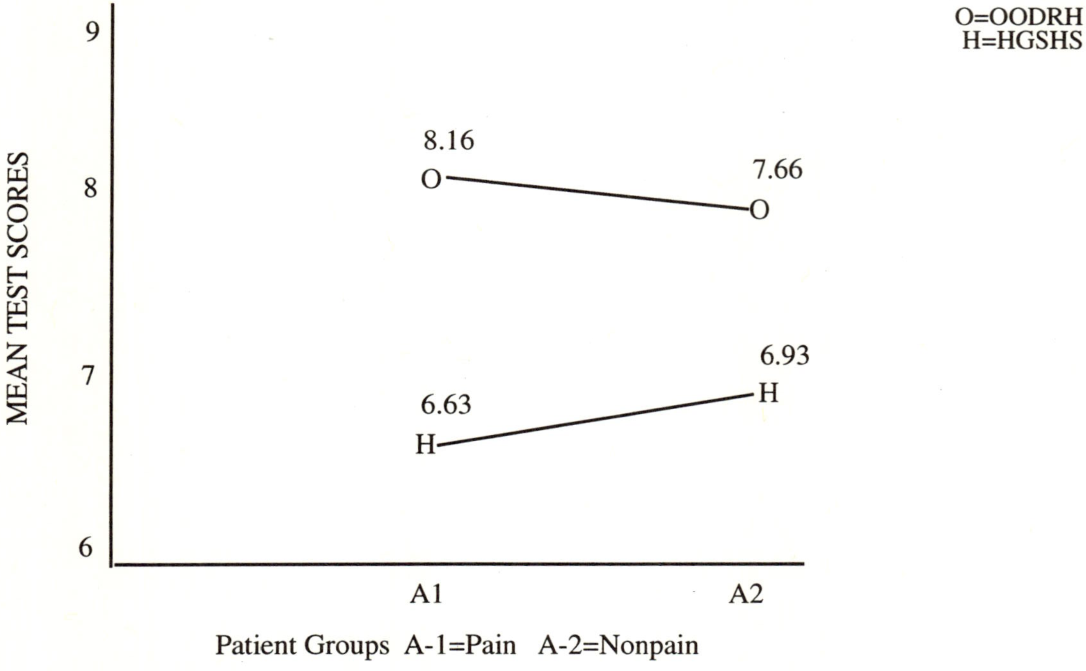

Figure B-2. Plot of Interaction between OODRH and HGSHS Scales

Table B–3. Analysis of Variance: Hypnosis Susceptibility Scales

Source	Sum of Squares	Degrees of Freedom	Mean of Squares	F	Required F
Between Groups (A)	1.70	1	1.70	.04	4052.00
Between Tests (B)	26.37	1	26.37	4.80	6.84
Interaction (A x B)	38.19	1	38.19	6.96	6.84
Within Sets (Error)	703.22	128	5.49		
Total	703.48	131			

Table B–4. Coefficients of Biserial Correlation:
Hypnotic Scales and Patient Groups

Variables	Pain Group	Standard Error of Correlation	Non-Pain Patients	Standard Error of Correlation
HGSHS	.377	.284	-.263	.268
OODRH	.696*	.284	.921*	.268

*Significantly correlated at <.05 level

it can be said that in this clinical setting the two scales are not reliably different. However, the interaction between the scales and the groups (see Table B–3 and Figure B–3) do show a significant difference. With a significant difference in the interaction, a further analysis was made to compare the HGSHS:A and the DRH as to their relative correlation in both pain and nonpain groups. The results of the biserial correlation comparison (Table B–4) show the DRH to have a significant positive correlated effect at less than the .05 level to treatment results of both the pain and the nonpain patient groups. The biserial correlation results showed the HGSHS:A to have no significant correlated effect to either group when compared to either pain or nonpain patient groups.

This study, therefore, found no significant difference in overall test scores for the two groups of patients defined as pain and nonpain patients. The results show that in this hypnotherapy-clinic setting, there tends to be a positive correlation between the scores of the DRH and the treatment results from the use of hypnotherapy, whereas no positive correlation was seen between the HGSHS:A scores and the treatment results. The correlation between the HGSHS:A and the DRH test results are poor by any standard for this clinical research.

DISCUSSION

This statistical study was conducted in an effort to investigate a correlation, or lack thereof, between a laboratory scale for hypnotizability and an observer estimate scale of depth of hypnosis in a clinical setting. It was stimulated by the belief of many clinicians that clinical patients seem to be much more hypnotizable than laboratory subjects. It utilized well-established laboratory tests for hypnosis susceptibility. Although the Orne-O'Connell Scale originated in the laboratory, it actually measures the subjects' reactions in the *state* of hypnosis, including the appearance and subjective experience of the patient during hypnosis and on being dehypnotized, and the actions during the early posthypnotic period. Since many clinicians have accepted the predicability of scales, it had been assumed that a patient who tested *low* for hypnosis susceptibility was not a candidate for the clinical tool of hypnosis. The present analysis of these statistics tends strongly to imply otherwise.

THE CLINICAL QUOTIENT

To help explain this difference between clinical and experimental hypnosis, the term *clinical quotient* is used. The authors do not doubt the validity of the laboratory tests. They do doubt the relevance of those tests to the clinical setting where the added important variables seem to include health, motivation, the transference, preparation of the patient, personalities of the therapist and the patient, the setting for the treatment, and the patient's previous concepts about hypnosis, among others.

POSSIBILITIES FOR FUTURE CLINICAL RESEARCH

The present project should be viewed as an initial attempt to approach the clinical and experimental situation critically. It is respectfully suggested that this be replicated with several additions. First, it should not be done as a gathering of a set of statistics waiting to be studied, but as an organized investigation. The HGSHS:A should be done not only before the treatment begins but after as well. This would also help establish whether the experience of success or failure in treatment caused this scale to be modified in the patients in question. Additionally, independent observers should be used to assess the DRH scores preferably at the first hypnosis as well as at the last. Independent observers should also assess the treatment results. It is also possible that other approaches to the statistical examinations would be of benefit in this type of project. The results are so marked that it is hoped that others will investigate the validity of the findings as well as note the clinical quotient as a reason for not relying on susceptibility tests only in utilizing this very valuable tool of clinical hypnosis.

Genuis (1995) recounts one of nine studies using a comparison of the results between high and low hypnotizability. There did not seem to be a relationship of this factor with the results of hypnotherapy. Genuis attributes this to flaws in the research (Wall and Womack 1989). I believe that our findings place his criticism in question. The laboratory test results do not correlate with clinical results, in our experience. He also describes the project by Katz and colleagues (1897) as using a within-hypnosis observation as correlating well with results. It was unfortunate that one of the susceptibility scales was not used.

APPENDIX B REFERENCES

Bentler, P., and Hilgard, E. (1963). A comparison of group and individual induction of hypnosis with self-scoring and observer-scoring. *International Journal of Clinical and Experimental Hypnosis* 11:49–54.

Bentler, P., and Roberts, M. (1963). Hypnotic susceptibility assessed in large groups. *International Journal of Clinical and Experimental Hypnosis* 11:93–97.

Bernheim, H. (1957). *Suggestive Therapeutics: A Treatise on the Nature and Uses of Hypnotism,* trans. C. H. Herter and G. P. Putnam. Westport, CT: Associated Book Sellers (Original work published 1889).

Braid, J. (1843). *Neuropnology, or the Rationale of Nervous Sleep Considered in Relation with Animal Magnetism.* New York: Arno.

Charcot, J. (1962). In *Psychology in the Making: Histories of Selected Research Problems,* ed. L. Postman. New York: Knopf.

Elifson, K., Runion, R., and Haber, A. (1982). *Fundamentals of Social Statistics.* Menlow Park, CA: Addison-Wesley.

Evans, F. J., and Schmeidler, D. (1966). Relationship between the Harvard Group Scale of Hypnotic Susceptibility and the Stanford Hypnotic Susceptibility Scale: Form C. *International Journal of Clinical and Experimental Hypnosis* 14:333–343.

Frankel, F. H., Apfel, R. J., Kelly, S. F., et al. (1979). The use of hypnotizability scales in the clinic: a review after six years. *International Journal of Clinical and Experimental Hypnosis* 27:63–73.

Genuis, M. L. (1995). Use of hypnosis in helping cancer patients control anxiety, pain and emesis: a review of recent empirical studies. *American Journal of Clinical Hypnosis* 37:316–325.

Gruenewald, D. (1982). Problems of relevance in the application of laboratory data to clinical situations. *International Journal of Clinical and Experimental Hypnosis* 30:345–353.

Hilgard, E. R. (1969). Pain as a puzzle for psychology and physiology. *American Psychologist* 24:103–113.

Hilgard, J. R. (1965). Hypnotic susceptibility and implications for measurement. *International Journal of Clinical and Experimental Hypnosis* 30:394–403.

——— (1979). *Personality and Hypnosis: A Study of Imaginative Involvement,* 2nd ed. Chicago: University of Chicago Press.

Hilgard, J. R., and Hilgard, E. R. (1979). Assessing hypnotic responsiveness in a clinical setting: a multi-item clinical scale and its advantages over single-item scales. *International Journal of Clinical and Experimental Hypnosis* 27:134–150.

Hilgard, J. R., and LeBaron, S. (1982). Relief of anxiety and pain in children and adolescents with cancer: Quantitative measures and clinical observations. *International Journal of Clinical and Experimental Hypnosis* 30:417–442.

Huck, S., Cormeir, W., and Boundes, W. (1974). *Reading Statistics and Research.* New York: Harper and Row.

Katz, E., Kellerman, J., and Ellenberg, L. (1987). Hypnosis in the reduction of acute pain and distress in children with cancer. *Journal of Pediatric Psychology* 12:379–394.

Kihlstrom, J. F., Diaz, W. A., McClellan, G. E., et al. (1980). Personality correlates of hypnotic susceptibility: needs for achievement and autonomy, self-monitoring and masculinity–femininity. *Americal Journal of Clinical and Experimental Hypnosis* 22:225–229.

Kroger, W. S. (1977). *Clinical and Experimental Hypnosis,* 2nd ed. Philadelphia: J.B. Lippincott.

Levitt, E. E., and Overley, T. M. (1965). Experience of the

hypnotist as a factor in hypnotic behavior. *International Journal of Clinical and Experimental Hypnosis* 13:34–38.

Meares, A. A. (1961). *A System of Medical Hypnosis.* Philadelphia: Saunders.

O'Connell, D. N., Orne, M. T., and Shor, R. E. (1966). A comparison of hypnotic susceptibility as assessed by diagnostic ratings and initial standardized test scores. *International Journal of Clinical and Experimental Hypnosis* 14:324–332.

Orne, M. T. (1966). Hypnosis, motivation and compliance. *American Journal of Psychiatry* 122.

Orne, M. T., and O'Connell, D. N. (1967). Diagnostic ratings of hypnotizability. *International Journal of Clinical and Experimantal Hypnosis* 115:125–133.

Perry, C., Gelfand, R., and Marcovitch, P. (1979). The relevance of hypnotic susceptibility in the clinical context. *Journal of Abnormal Psychology* 88:592–603.

Sacerdote, P. (1982). Techniques of hypnotic intervention with pain patients. In *Psychological Approaches to the Management of Pain,* eds. J. Barber, and C. Adrian. New York: Brunner/ Mazel.

Sarbin, T. R. (1962). Attempts to understand hypnotic phenomena. In *Psychology in the Making: Histories of Selected Research Problems,* ed. I. Postman. New York: Knopf.

Schafer, D. W. (1980). *The five states of hypnosis.* Presented at the Annual Scientific Meeting of the Society for Clinical and Experimental Hypnosis, Chicago.

Shor, R. E. (1969). Hypnosis and the concept of generalized reality orientation. Three dimensions of hypnotic depth. In *Altered States of Consciousness,* ed. C. T. Tart, pp. 233–250; 251–261. New York: Wiley.

Shor, R. E., and Orne, E. C. (1963). Norms on the Harvard Group Scale of Hypnotic Susceptibility, Form A. *International Journal of Clinical Hypnosis* 11:47–49.

Tart, C. T. (1979). Measuring the depth of an altered state of consciousness, with particular reference to self-report scales of hypnotic depth. In *Hypnosis: Developments in Research and New Perspectives,* ed. E. Fromm, and R. E. Shor. New York: Aldine.

Wadden, T. A., and Anderton, C. H. (1981). The clinical use of hypnosis. *Psychological Bulletin* 91:215–243.

Wall, V., and Womack, W. (1989). Hypnotic versus active cognitive strategies for alleviation of procedural distress in pediatric oncology patients. *American Journal of Clinical Hypnosis* 31:181–191.

Weitzenhoffer, M. M., and Hilgard, E. R. (1959). *Stanford Hypnotic Susceptibility Scale: Form A and B.* Palo Alto, CA: Consulting Psychologist Press.

REFERENCES

Alexander, A. S. (1986). The pain of acute gout. *American Journal of Medicine* 80:(suppl 3A):133.

Alexander, F. (1950). *Psychosomatic Medicine.* New York: W. W. Norton.

American Psychiatric Association. *Diagnostic and Statistical Manual IV.* (1994). Washington, DC: American Psychiatric Association.

Araoz, D. L. (1985). *The New Hypnosis.* New York: Brunner/Mazel.

Barber, J. (1982). Incorporating hypnosis in the management of chronic pain. In *Psychological Approaches to the Management of Pain,* ed. J. Barber, and C. Adrian. New York: Brunner/Mazel.

Benson, H. (1975). *The Relaxation Response.* New York: Morrow.

Bowers, K. S. (1976). *Hypnosis for the Seriously Curious.* New York: W. W. Norton.

Cannon, W. B. (1929). *Bodily Changes in Pain, Hunger, Fear and Rage.* Boston: Branford.

Cheek, D. B. (1959). Unconscious perception of meaningful sounds during surgical anesthesia as revealed under hypnosis. *American Journal of Clinical Hypnosis* 1:101–113.

Cheek, D. B., and LeCron, L. M. (1968). *Clinical Hypnotherapy.* New York: Grune & Stratton.

Cornelius, R., and Schneider, H. J. (1988). Gouty arthritis in the adult. *Radiology Clinics of North America* 26:1267–1276.

Coue, E. (1923). *How to Practice Suggestion and Autosuggestion.* New York: American Library Service.

Crasilneck, H. B. (1995). The use of the Crasilneck bombardment technique in problems of intractable organic pain. *American Journal of Clinical Hypnosis* 37:255–266.

Crue, B. L. (1975). *Pain: Research and Treatment.* New York: Academic Press.

Engel, G. L. (1959). Psychogenic pain and the pain-prone patient. *American Journal of Medicine* 26:899–918.

Erickson, M. H. (1959). Childhood hypnosis. *American Journal of Clinical Hypnosis* 2:3–21. Reprinted in the *Collected Papers of Milton H. Erickson,* vol. 1, ed. Ernest L. Rossi. New York: Holsted Press.

____ (1966). The interspersal hypnotic technique for symptom correction and pain control. *Americal Journal of Clinical Hypnosis* 8:198–209.

Ewin, D. M. (1976). Preventing third degree burns. International Congress on Hypnosis, Philadelphia.

____ (1980). Constant pain syndrome: its psychological meaning and cure using hypnoanalysis in clinical hypnosis. In *Clinical Hypnosis in Medicine,* ed. H. J. Wain. Chicago, London: Year Book Medical.

____ (1986). Emergency room hypnosis for the burned patient. *American Journal of Clinical Hypnosis* 29:7–12.

Ferenczi, S. (1955). *Selected Papers of Sandor Ferenczi,* ed. M. Balint. New York: Basic Books.

Fordyce, W. (1976). *Behavioral Methods for Chronic Pain and Illness.* St. Louis: C. V. Mosby.

Freedman, D. X. (1992). The search: body, mind, and human purpose. *American Journal of Psychiatry* 149(7)858–866.

Gabbard, G. O. (1992). Psychodynamic psychiatry in the "decade of the brain." *American Journal of Psychiatry* 149(8)991–1010.

Gardner, G. G., and Olness, K. (1981). *Hypnosis and Hypnotherapy with Children.* New York: Grune & Stratton.

Genuis, M. L. (1995). The use of hypnosis in helping cancer patients control anxiety, pain, and emesis: a review of recent empirical studies. *American Journal of Clinical Hypnosis* 37:316–325.

Hart, D. F. (1983). Gout and non-gout through the ages. *British Journal of Clinical Practice* 39:91–92.

Hilgard, E. R. (1975). Hypnosis in the relief of pain. In *The Control of Pain,* ed. M. Weisenberg. New York: Psychological Dimensions.

——— (1977). *Divided Consciousness Multiple Controls in Human Thought and Action.* New York: John Wiley.

Hilgard, E. R., and Hilgard, J. R. (1975). *Hypnotic Susceptibility.* New York: Harcourt, Brace & World.

——— (1994). *Hypnosis in the Relief of Pain,* 2nd ed. Los Altos, CA: William Kaufmann.

Hilgard, J. R., and LeBaron, S. (1984). *Hypnotherapy of Pain in Children with Cancer.* Los Altos, CA: William Kaufmann.

Joranson, D. E. (1995). Intractable pain treatment laws and regulations. *Bulletin of the American Pain Society* 5:1–3, 15–17.

Krane, E. J., and Heller, L. B. (1995). The prevalence of phantom sensation and pain in pediatric amputees. *Journal of Pain and Symptom Management* 10:21–29.

Kroger, W. S. (1973). Acupunctural analgesia: its explanation by conditioning theory, autogenic training and hypnosis. *American Journal of Psychiatry* 138:855.

____ (1977). *Clinical and Experimental Hypnosis,* 2nd ed. Philadelphia: J. B. Lippincott.

Le Page, K. E., and Schafer, D. W. (1994). Unilateral lachrymation associated with somatic memory of pain. *Hypnos* 21:238–245.

Livingston, W. K. (1943). *Pain Mechanisms and Stress.* New York: Macmillan. (Note: There is a 1976 edition with a forward by Ronald Melzack, published in New York by Plenum.)

Lynn, S., and Rhue, J. W., eds. (1991). *Theories of Hypnosis: Current Models and Perspectives.* New York: Guilford.

Melzack, R. (1975). The McGill pain questionaire: major properties and scoring methods. *Pain* 11:85–92.

Melzack, R., and Wall, P. D. (1965). Pain mechanisms: a new theory. *Science* 150:971–979.

____ (1983). *The Challenge of Pain.* New York: Basic Books.

Merskey, H., and Bogduk, N. (1994). *Classification of Chronic Pain,* 2nd ed. Seattle: IASP Press.

Milne, G. (1995). Hypnotic treatment for stress-induced trigeminal neuralgia. *Hypnos* 22:39–41.

Olness, K. (1981). Imagery (self hypnosis) as adjunct therapy in childhood cancer: clinical experiences with 25 patients. *Journal of Clinical Hematology/Oncology* 3:313–321.

____ (1989). Hypnotherapy: a cyberphysiologic strategy in pain management. *Pediatric Clinics of North America* 36:873–884.

Orne, M. T., and O'Connell, D. N. (1967). Diagnostic rating of hypnotizability. *International Journal of Clinical and Experimental Hypnosis* 15:125–133.

Pace, J. B. (1976). *Pain: A Personal Experience.* Chicago: Nelson-Hall.

Pavlov, I. (1928). *Lectures on Conditioned Reflexes.* New York: Liveright.

Roark, A. (1991). The accelerated search for relief from pain. *Los Angeles Times,* October 28.

Rossi, E. L., and Cheek, D. B. (1988). *Mind-Body Therapy: Methods of Ideodynamic Healing in Hypnosis.* New York: Norton.

Sacerdote, P. (1966). The uses of hypnosis in cancer patients. *Annals of the New York Academy of Science* 125:1011–1019.

_____ (1970). Theory and practice of pain control in malignancy and other protracted or recurring painful illnesses. *International Journal of Clinical and Experimental Hypnosis* 18:160–180.

Schafer, D. W. (1966). The bizarre misuse of medication in pseudoneurotic schizophrenia. *Psychosomatics* 7:376–381.

_____ (1975). Hypnosis use on a burn unit. *International Journal of Clinical and Experimental Hypnosis* 23:1–14.

_____ (1981). The recognition and hypnotherapy of patients with unrecognized altered states. *American Journal of Clinical Hypnosis* 23:176–183.

_____ (1984a). The management of pain in the cancer patient. *Comprehensive Therapy* 10:41–45.

_____ (1984b). Pain, emotions and the cancer patient. *Surgical Annals* 16:57–67.

_____ (1984c). Beware of the hypnoquacks. *Orange County Medical Association Bulletin,* June, pp. 25–36.

_____ (1986). Recognizing multiple personality patients. *American Journal of Psychotherapy* 40:500–510.

_____ (1989). Hypnosis: a tool for diagnosis. *Hypnos: Swedish Journal of Clinical and Experimental Hypnosis* 16:19–24.

_____ (1994a). *A psychiatrist views cancer and hypnosis.* Presented at the 36th Annual Scientific Meeting of the American Society of Clinical Hypnosis, Philadelphia.

_____ (1994b). *A psychiatrist looks at auto-immunity, a preliminary report.* Presented at the 13th International Congress of hypnosis, Melbourne, Australia.

Schafer, D. W., and Hernandez, A. (1978). Hypnosis, pain and the context of therapy. *International Journal of Clinical and Experimental Hypnosis* 3:143–153.

Shafer, T. A. (1962). Hypnosis in the management and control of trigeminal neuralgia: two case reports. *American Journal of Clinical Hypnosis* 5:138.

Simonton, O. C., Matthews, S. S., and Creighton, J. (1978). *Getting Well Again.* Los Angeles: J. P. Tarscher.

Sternbach, R. A. (1974). *Pain Patients: Traits and Treatment.* New York: Academic Press.

Swanson, D. W. (1984). Chronic pain as a third pathological emotion. *American Journal of Psychiatry* 141:210–214.

Szasz, T. S. (1957). *Pain and Pleasure: A Study of Bodily Feelings.* New York: Basic Books.

Travell, J. G., and Simons, D. G. (1983/1992). *The Trigger Point Manual: Myofascial Pain and Dysfunction,* vol. 1 and 2. Baltimore: Williams & Wilkins.

Tsuchiya, N., and Williams, R. C., Jr. (1992). Molecular mimicry: hypothesis or reality? *Western Journal of Medicine* 157:133–138.

Van Hagen, K. O. (1956). Chronic intolerable pain. *Journal of the American Medical Association.*

Watkins H. H. (1980). The selected abreaction. *International Journal of Clinical and Experimental Hypnosis* 28:101–113.

Watkins, J. G. (1971). The affect bridge: a hypnoanalytic technique. *International Journal of Clinical and Experimental Hypnosis* 19:21–27.

Watkins, J. G., and Watkins, H. H. (1990). Dissociation and displacement, where goes the ouch? *American Journal of Clinical Hypnosis* 33:1.

Weitzenhoffer, A. M., and Hilgard, E. H. (1959). *Stanford Hypnotic Susceptibility Scale: Forms A and B.* Palo Alto, CA: Consulting Psychologists Press.

Wicks, G. (1984). *The somatic bridge.* Personal communication.

INDEX